Stop Overeating
for Good

Stop Overeating for Good

Overcome Food Obsession
with Dr. Prasad's Proven Program

Balasa L. Prasad, M.D.

with Catherine Whitney

Avery   a member of Penguin Group (USA) Inc.   New York

Published by the Penguin Group

Penguin Group (USA) Inc., 375 Hudson Street, New York, New York 10014, USA •
Penguin Group (Canada), 90 Eglinton Avenue East, Suite 700, Toronto, Ontario M4P 2Y3,
Canada (a division of Pearson Penguin Canada Inc.) • Penguin Books Ltd, 80 Strand,
London WC2R 0RL, England • Penguin Ireland, 25 St Stephen's Green, Dublin 2, Ireland
(a division of Penguin Books Ltd) • Penguin Group (Australia), 250 Camberwell Road,
Camberwell, Victoria 3124, Australia (a division of Pearson Australia Group Pty Ltd) •
Penguin Books India Pvt Ltd, 11 Community Centre, Panchsheel Park, New Delhi–110 017,
India • Penguin Group (NZ), Cnr Airborne and Rosedale Roads, Albany, Auckland 1310,
New Zealand (a division of Pearson New Zealand Ltd) • Penguin Books (South Africa)
(Pty) Ltd, 24 Sturdee Avenue, Rosebank, Johannesburg 2196, South Africa

Penguin Books Ltd, Registered Offices: 80 Strand, London WC2R 0RL, England

ISBN 1-58333-268-5

Printed in the United States of America
1   3   5   7   9   10   8   6   4   2

Book design by Meighan Cavanaugh

Neither the publisher nor the authors are engaged in rendering professional advice or services
to the individual reader. The ideas, procedures, and suggestions contained in this book are not
intended as a substitute for consulting with your physician. All matters regarding your health
require medical supervision. Neither the authors nor the publisher shall be liable or responsible
for any loss or damage allegedly arising from any information or suggestion in this book.

Most Avery books are available at special quantity discounts for bulk purchase for sales
promotions, premiums, fund-raising, and educational needs. Special books or book excerpts
also can be created to fit specific needs. For details, write Penguin Group (USA) Inc. Special
Markets, 375 Hudson Street, New York, NY 10014.

While the authors have made every effort to provide accurate telephone numbers and
Internet addresses at the time of publication, neither the publisher nor the authors assume
any responsibility for errors, or for changes that occur after publication. Further, the publisher
does not have any control over and does not assume any responsibility for author or third-
party websites or their content.

This book is dedicated with love and gratitude to:

My parents, especially my mother. She was an extraordinary woman who instilled in me discipline, compassion, and a deep sense of responsibility. She taught me to dream big and work hard to make that dream a reality. She encouraged me to believe in myself and to do the best I could with my God-given talents.

My wife, Vashantha, who is the love of my life. She has always been a great inspiration for me—highly supportive, constantly encouraging me to work hard and to be proud of everything I do in my profession. She truly is a life partner at home and at work.

My daughter and only child, Bindu, a smart, wonderful young lady who has been my greatest fan and best critic. Bindu has always helped me with remarkable comments and suggestions.

They say that there is a woman behind every successful man, but in my case I feel blessed to have had three smart and intuitive women who have helped me to come this far in life.

ACKNOWLEDGMENTS

Special thanks to Judge Judy Sheindlin. She believed in my work, and encouraged me to write this important series. Judy is one of the most intelligent and astute individuals whom I have had the pleasure of meeting.

Endless thanks to Catherine Whitney, who thoroughly understood my philosophical and scientific approach in dealing with habits. She literally transformed my manuscript into an interesting and enlightening book. She is a wonderful writer, and I feel very lucky to have had the opportunity to work with her.

My thanks to my literary agents, Jane Dystel and Miriam Goderich, who took an early interest in my work, and who always believed in me. They worked tirelessly to see that my book found the right publishing home.

My editors at Avery/Penguin, Megan Newman and Lucia Watson, have showed enthusiasm and creativity, and I am proud to have them behind my work. It was Megan who decided to present the material in a series of practical books in order to spread their impact as far as possible. Lucia has shepherded this book through the process with great sensitivity to my intentions.

Thanks to Dr. Preetham Grandhi, a child and adolescent psychiatrist, who engaged me in a healthy debate about psychiatric views. I am also grateful to the nursing staff at Mount Vernon Hospital, who served as my spokespeople to my patients and the public. They are, and will always be, my biggest cheerleaders.

Last but not least, I want to thank my patients of the past twenty-five years, who have helped me to strengthen my beliefs and my profound philosophy. They have taught me firsthand that there are no simple answers to life's complex problems. It is very gratifying for me to know that I have been of help to them in dealing with challenges in their day-to-day lives, and that I have played a part in their happiness, health, and success.

CONTENTS

Part One

The Mind
of an Overeater

1

The Craving Beyond Food

I BEGAN MY PRACTICE treating patients with addictions to smoking, alcohol, and drugs. I didn't always consider overeating an addictive activity. In fact, my attitude about overeating and obesity was that it was a simple matter of choice. After all, it had not been difficult for me to maintain the same weight throughout my adult life. I did not take extraordinary measures to keep my caloric needs in balance. It seemed like the most simple equation: eat more calories than you expend, and you will gain weight.

If you think my previous attitude sounds arrogant and insulting to the millions of people who struggle with weight problems, you would be right. But it took a forty-five-year-old female patient to straighten me out. She helped me realize how insensitive and ignorant I was about a serious problem.

When Rachel* arrived at my office and informed me that

*Names have been changed to protect the privacy of my patients.

she wanted help losing forty pounds, I was curious about why she came to me. "If you want to lose weight, you need a dietician," I said. "You've come to the wrong place."

Rachel was ready with a response. "Dr. Prasad, why do you treat people for alcoholism, drug abuse, and smoking?"

Without hesitation, I replied that people with these problems need special help because they are addicted to the substances in question.

"Well, I'm addicted, too," Rachel said firmly. "I'm a food junkie. Just like your smoker or alcoholic, I have vowed hundreds of times to stop devouring fattening foods, but I always go back. I feel as if I can't help it. Isn't that the definition of an addict?"

I was intrigued. "Tell me about your compulsion," I said. "You've piqued my interest."

Rachel described a daily pattern that revolved around food. Each morning, she awoke with a determination to eat in moderation and resist junk food, but as the day went on her resolve faded. There was always a trigger. Sometimes it would be an afternoon gabfest with friends, which was incomplete without food and drink. A restaurant meal with her husband would include platters of savory foods, which she found irresistible. Relaxing in the evenings, she would snack through her favorite television shows. Usually, by 10:00 P.M., Rachel's bloated stomach was begging for mercy and crying out for her to stop stuffing her mouth. But instead of heeding her stomach's pleas, she would continue to pacify her palate until she went to bed. The next morning, Rachel would stare at her figure in the mirror, feeling disgusted, and would begin the day with another empty promise to eat less.

After describing her pattern, Rachel looked me in the eye and asked, "Do you still think I need no outside help to control my eating habit? Do you really believe that a dietician is the answer?"

I chuckled a little. Rachel had tricked me into seeing her problem in a different context. She did me a great favor that day, by helping me open my mind to the plight of obese patients. I took her on, and in the course of two years helped her to lose forty pounds, using the same principles that I have found to be effective with addicts. We began with an examination of her life.

Rachel described herself as basically a happy-go-lucky, pleasant, compassionate person with lots of spunk. She had met her husband, John, in college, and they fell in love and married after graduation. She worked hard for two years, and then quit her job when she got pregnant. Rachel loved being a mother, and within three years she had two young children who kept her on her toes.

As Rachel happily involved herself in the lives of her children, her husband was prospering in business: he worked long hours and traveled frequently, but this did not bother Rachel too much while the kids consumed her attention. Things changed when her second child started college and Rachel found herself alone in the house without any purpose to her days.

To kill the boredom, Rachel started to read novels while snacking on cookies, candy, and chips. When reading grew tiring, she started meeting her friends for lunch or drinks in the afternoon. The pounds kept creeping on, and she resolved to join a health club or go to a spa, but she never went through with it. Basically, she was so ashamed of her appearance, that she didn't want to be seen in a health club. Besides, she had no strong motivation to lose weight because her husband didn't seem at all bothered by her appearance. This went on for a couple of years, until Rachel could not stand herself any longer. "I was told you could fix food addictions," she told me. "I'm ready."

I smiled at her. "I'm not a fixer," I said, "but I may be able to help you."

Rachel considered her overwhelming craving for food as a force outside herself that she could not control. She was wrong. Her craving came from within. It came from the empty place of a life without purpose, and the compulsion to fill her emptiness with food. Only when Rachel changed her life—returning to school and finding a new profession as a home decorator—was she able to change her eating behavior.

So, was Rachel a food addict? How can eating be an addiction? After all, we need food to live. In the years since I treated Rachel, I have seen many patients with similar stories. They all list the diets they have tried, and often tell me that they have lost and regained hundreds of pounds in their lifetimes. Whenever they diet, they are consumed with thoughts of the foods they can no longer have. They are not happy campers. Eventually, they return to their former eating habits. Statistics show that more than 90 percent of all diets fail over the long term.

Why are the statistics so discouraging? People who embark on rigorous diet programs are highly motivated to succeed. They want to be healthy. They want to look slim and fit and have the bodies others see as attractive. They have enormous self-control in the short term. They struggle and sacrifice and deprive themselves in order to meet their goals. But when they "fall off the wagon" and resume their old patterns, they feel as helpless as an addict who craves a shot of heroin.

Food, as a substance, cannot realistically be compared to mind-altering drugs like heroin and cocaine. Nor can its effects be likened to those triggered by alcohol or nicotine. The addictive pull of food is constructed in the mind. It cannot be objectified. There is not a diet in existence that can eliminate the craving for food. That's because the craving is not caused by food. It is the result of an emotional need. Until the emotional need is exposed and addressed, all the diets in the world will not help.

One problem with our notion of food addiction is that we equate addiction with helplessness. And the simple truth of the matter is that no one is helpless to control food intake. That's the cheap and easy way out, a justification that is built on lies. You are not helpless against your craving for food. The only requirement is that you be willing to face the truth about what is really driving your compulsion.

A Bitter Hunger

Janet stepped off the scale in my office and turned away. "Don't tell me the number," she said hurriedly. Her face was flushed and she looked ready to burst into tears. I led her into my office and offered her a seat.

"You seem quite upset," I said gently. "Try to relax." She sat, taking deep breaths to calm her nerves.

Janet was a twenty-three-year-old accountant who carried 275 pounds on a five-foot-three frame. When she made the appointment, she'd said she was desperate to get her weight under control. Now she seemed unsure that she wanted to be there.

"I'm curious," I said. "Why didn't you want to know the number on the scale?"

Janet sighed. "Every time I get weighed it has a terrible effect on me," she said. "Look, Dr. Prasad, I know I'm fat. You know I'm fat. What's the point of belaboring it? Getting on the scale feels like a big insult."

Janet went on to describe the programs she'd tried, such as

Weight Watchers and Overeaters Anonymous. "The first thing they make you do is get on the scale, and then they want to talk about that awful number," she said. "Talking about it just makes me feel worse, and that causes me to eat more." She confessed miserably that after a weigh-in she usually went home and ate voraciously. Then she felt guilty and angry with herself.

"I can't stand to be reminded of my weight," Janet told me. "It's been years since I've stood in front of a full-length mirror. I'm afraid that seeing myself will upset me and trigger another binge." She laughed bitterly. "If I went to a fat farm, I'd probably be the only one who would weigh more at the end of the course than I did at the beginning. Dr. Prasad, I have tried every diet, every pill, everything, and I always fail. I have tried to resign myself to being fat—to accept myself the way I am—but I can't get over feeling betrayed."

Ah, I thought. Now we were getting somewhere. "Tell me more about that," I said. "Why do you feel betrayed?"

"How else should I feel?" she asked. "I've done everything I could do, and my body refuses to cooperate. It's not fair that I have this body to begin with. My sister and brother both take after my father, who is tall and lean. I had to take after my fat mother. It's so unfair."

"You feel cheated," I said, understanding. "You think you got a bum deal from birth."

Janet shrugged. "Didn't I? If I had been born with my sister's body, I wouldn't be sitting here today."

As we continued talking, I discovered that the unfairness of life was a central theme for Janet. At one point she was telling me about the mechanic she'd been dating for two years and how their love life was nothing to brag about. She said that her boyfriend had never commented on her appearance and never encouraged her to lose weight. Suddenly, she made a strange comment: "If I were Oprah Winfrey, I, too, could have easily controlled my eating and lost all the extra weight."

For a moment, I was taken aback by the sudden shift in the direction of our conversation. One moment Janet was talking about her boyfriend, and in the next moment she was talking about Oprah Winfrey. I asked Janet why she would have an easier time losing weight if she were Oprah. "Oprah didn't exactly have an easy time of it," I said. "She tried and failed many times to lose weight."

"But she finally made it," Janet said. "Look, I'm sure I'd be able to do it, too, if I could snap my fingers and have a team of trainers and nutritionists at my beck and call—not to mention a personal chef."

Everywhere she turned, Janet saw examples of the unfairness of life that became the excuses for her situation. Why wasn't she born with her sister's body? Why wasn't she born Oprah Winfrey? Why, why, why?

Unfortunately, it is a bitter, irrevocable truth that no one will be able to set foot on the winning path as long as they feel that they have been shortchanged by nature and unfairly treated by the world. The will to change must come from within.

"Let's consider Oprah Winfrey," I suggested. "First of all, she wasn't always the big star she is today. Second, she was a phenomenal success before she put a dent in her weight issue. Even though she had all of the advantages of power and wealth, for many years she remained unable to conquer her weight problem. What happened to transform her? Was it more money? More fame? Not at all. It was the decision, backed up by action, to become healthy and fit forever. She invested her energy and time to make it a reality. In other words, first she changed her attitude, and then she changed her weight. The Oprah you envy today is not where she is because of fame, money, or a team of trainers and nutritionists. She is there because of her determination to remain fit and healthy that made it possible for her to take control of her weight problem. The day she loses that determination to remain fit is the day she will not have the patience or discipline to maintain her healthy weight."

I leaned across the desk and looked into her hurt eyes. "Janet," I said, "I am going to tell you the truth. You may not like it or understand it, but if you accept this truth, you will overcome your eating problem."

She sat up eagerly. "Tell me."

"Your problem is not your inability to eat right," I said. "Nor is it being born with a body that tends toward fat. Your problem—the thing that is stopping you from succeeding—is your feeling of bitterness and betrayal. Get to the bottom of that and put it to rest, and the weight will melt off."

Janet stared at me like I was nuts. In that respect she wasn't much different from most patients who come to me for help with their addictions or compulsions. Confused and ashamed of their inability to control their behavior, they conclude that the matter is out of their hands. Like Janet, they blame their genes, or their circumstances, or their mixed-up brain chemicals. They don't think they are normal, and they envy the people around them who seem to so easily take life in stride without the crutches on which they rely. They speak of an insatiable craving, as if a demon lived inside them that they could not expunge.

This is the predicament Janet faced as she sat in my office. "You cannot make any progress as long as your self-esteem is shot and you feel embittered by your plight," I told her. "If you truly want to stop overeating, you must first get rid of the negative emotions that are driving your behavior."

Janet was perplexed by this statement. She thought I had it backward. "If I don't overeat, I'll feel better about myself," she said.

"There's the rub," I replied. "For many years, you have assumed that your low self-esteem and anger were a result of your inability to control your eating and your weight. You have tried to diet, but that has only made you feel worse, and made your problem greater. I am offering you a different approach: develop a positive regard for yourself first, and the overeating will stop. In other words, change your *mind* about yourself, the world, and your eating, and your habit will change, too."

Living to Eat

Every human being is born with the potential to develop addictions or insatiable cravings because we are inherently pleasure seekers. If you eliminate the constant fear for survival, which we have effectively done in most modern societies, the pursuit of pleasure becomes dominant. However, most people recognize that they must rein in their pleasure-seeking behaviors and approach them with moderation. This self-regulation becomes second nature for most of us. We do not have to struggle every minute to deny ourselves pleasure. If there is a quart of ice cream in the freezer, we can eat a serving without feeling an overwhelming urge to finish off the whole thing.

However, in the last fifty years, a remarkable shift has occurred in Western society regarding our attitudes and behaviors around food. The ordinary standards and restraints have all but disappeared. At some point we crossed the line from enjoyment to indulgence, and as a result food has lost its true identity as a source of nourishment. Most Americans cannot recognize hunger signals or evaluate their true nutritional needs. They supersize with abandon, whether they want or need large portions. Nearly every activity seems to be accompanied by food. People wander through malls eating. Food and drink concessions are more profitable than ticket sales at theaters and sports events. The explosive combination of the vendors' desire to make money and the consumers' desire to devour food has led to an overeating frenzy in most parts of this country. Meanwhile, we are sending our children the message that they must constantly be eating and drinking in order to be satisfied.

When pleasure is the predominant purpose of eating, food becomes a want and not a need. That's where we start on the slippery slope to addictive behavior. The more an individual is driven to derive pleasure or comfort from food, the more they want, and the more demanding their emotions become. Why not eat? The food is there, within easy reach, it's delicious and satisfying, it was made with love. You can savor its taste and texture and forget all of your troubles in the meantime. When the world is letting you down and stressing you out, you can curl up with a tasty snack and exact a sweet revenge.

Everyone understands this pleasure principle, and when it comes to food, there is very little stigma attached. Unlike mind-altering drugs or smoking, we are encouraged to eat, and sometimes even made to feel guilty if we don't partake. Refusal to accept food when it's offered to us brands us as unsociable, unappreciative, health nuts, or spoilsports. It has become second nature to equate food with emotional satisfaction. Ironically, at the same time we coax one another to eat, we shun people who are obese. It's a no-win situation.

If you are serious about your decision to stop overeating for good, you must be willing to make three commitments:

1. The commitment to change your attitude about the role that food plays in your life, and to sacrifice a certain amount of the pleasure you take in foods that do you harm.
2. The commitment to give up the habit of dieting to achieve short-term weight loss goals, and to face the truth that all weight-loss diets are shams that increase the emotional hold food has over you.
3. The commitment to take the steps I recommend to identify and address the emotional drive that triggers your eating behavior, and to stop overeating for good.

If you are willing to make that commitment, read on.

2

A Society in Denial

HUMAN NATURE never ceases to amaze me. Here we are, well on our way into the twenty-first century, capable of caressing the heavens with our satellites, space shuttles, and space stations. We have made it possible for ordinary people to reach out and touch their loved ones anywhere in the world through sophisticated communications technology. And yet we still have not mastered the simplest dictate of life: how to eat right. I don't think eating right is rocket science. Yet the diet and nutrition business in this country is enormous. Countless programs, books, studies, and companies are devoted to showing people how to eat right, and the advice is often in conflict or confusing. For example, experts once believed that a high-protein, low-carbohydrate diet was the best approach. Now that concept is outdated. At one time it was believed that only an extremely low-fat diet was healthy, but now a moderate amount of fat is recommended. It is currently in vogue to measure foods against the glycemic index, which is just a complicated, scientific-sounding way of telling people what they already know—high-fiber, whole foods are better than doughnuts! We are constantly feeling the need to trick ourselves with newly packaged terms and ideas—to reinvent the wheel with fancy names. The only thing this accomplishes is more confusion among laypeople, and more failure for the hapless dieter. Every season brings new diet theories, packaged in expensive books and tapes, often written by people who claim that they have found the true secret to weight loss that has eluded everyone else.

Even the government has gotten into the act, with poor results. In 1992, the U.S. Department of Agriculture (USDA) introduced the Food Pyramid in the hope that Americans would be able to understand and follow a simple concept in which foods were arranged in a linear order according to their quality and recommended daily intake. Yet in the years since the Food Pyramid was first introduced, the number of obese people in America has doubled, and the number of people suffering from diabetes, heart disease, strokes, and kidney disease has almost tripled. Current statistics reveal that only 35 percent of Americans are at their recommended weight. The other 65 percent are considered to be overweight, and one-third of these are considered obese.

According to one study, nine million children between the ages of five and sixteen are obese. The same study reveals that if these children eliminated one can of soda a day, they would lose fifteen pounds in one year. This is not a new idea. Yet soda machines abound in school cafeterias, and most children are resistant to the idea of drinking more water and fewer sugary drinks. In 1950, an average of eleven gallons of soda a year was consumed per child. In 2003, the average was forty-six gallons. This is in spite of our increased knowledge of nutrition, and the billions of dollars being spent by government and private agencies to address the obesity epidemic. Everyone knows drinking too much soda is unhealthy, but nobody wants to take the responsibility to change the trend. Parents blame soda manufacturers for not caring about children's health. Soda manufacturers, in return, blame nutritional scientists for not coming up with a healthy soda alternative without compromising on taste. Scientists blame government agencies for lack of research funds to develop the right mix of drinks for children. All of them are busy pointing fingers at each other instead of addressing the true issue. While this blame game goes in circles, children are getting fatter by the day.

Twenty million Americans suffer from type 2 diabetes, meaning that they are diabetic mainly by virtue of their weight. Another 50 million Americans are prediabetic. At this rate, we are on the way to being the fattest country on earth, if we have not already earned this distinction.

Nature's Truth

It is a simple truth that the food most appealing to the palate is least friendly to the body. Nature has been very clear about this message since the dawn of time. This rule applies not only to food but to other chemical substances, like meta-amphetamines (commonly known as methamphetamines), cocaine, heroin, and nicotine. These substances are very appealing to the mind, but incredibly dangerous to the body.

Americans may be intelligent, but we are not so smart. If we were, we would not try to twist nature's truth, because every time we have done so in the past, we have failed. Take the example of trans fats. Trans fats were first developed to meet the public demand for appealing texture and good taste, without the health hazards of saturated fats found in meat and butter. Trans fat, which is composed of partially hydrogenated vegetable oils, was supposed to allow people to have their cake and eat it too, but thirty years later it has been deemed so unhealthy that the USDA has now recommended that we cut down on our use. In 2005, New York City health officials decreed that all restaurants eliminate trans fats in their frying and instead use pure oils.

Nature does not offer a free pass. If you want to enjoy refined, delicious foods like barbecued ribs, doughnuts, and steamy, juicy, delicate lobster dipped in butter sauce, be prepared to pay a price down the line. There is no escape from nature's law.

The Myth of Rescue

Obesity as a result of overeating and lack of exercise has reduced the average life expectancy by four to nine months. That doesn't sound like much, but it's alarming that life expectancy should be decreasing at all. For most of this century, thanks to medical technology and better health habits, average life expectancy has been steadily on the rise. Yet according to the *New England Journal of Medicine,* our children will have a shorter life expectancy than their grandparents. The culprit is obesity. That fact should be a rude awakening for every parent.

But it's not just life expectancy that is suffering. Our unhealthy eating habits are also compromising our quality of life. We can see this all around us. While our advanced health-care technology may spare obese people from early death due to diabetes, heart disease, vascular disease, and kidney failure, the lifestyle of these individuals is nothing to brag about. Most of their time is spent in doctor's offices, hospitals, and pharmacies. They have little time or energy to work productively or enjoy satisfying lives.

For the last five years, I have questioned many obese people who have not yet suffered visible consequences about what they think will happen if they continue their current eating habits. For the most part, they haven't given the matter much thought. They don't think there is any urgency about changing their ways because they haven't had problems thus far. Usually, people tell me that they'd like to make some changes but it's just too hard. They love their food—what can they do? For these people, the much heralded advances in medical technology are actually a detriment to change, because they reinforce the myth of rescue. They assume that if they get sick they'll be rescued by a magic pill or a simple surgical procedure—liposuction, a vascular stent, gastric bypass. The idea that medical technology will save people from every conceivable health-related problem is promoted regularly in the media, with frequent reports on promising new procedures or medications that will reverse the damage done by lifetimes of overindulgent living. I am not denying that medical technology has come a long way in helping people. However, I believe that the public should be aware of the progress we have made and the limitations of the medical field.

We need a serious reality check. There is a lot of information available about the ill effects of overeating on the body, and tremendous advances in the health-care industry like heart, kidney, and bone marrow transplants, to help sick people. Unfortunately, the public is kept in the dark about the limitations of advanced technology. For instance, consider the kidney and vascular problems triggered by diabetes, which is very common in obese adults. These problems can be managed to sustain life through medications, dialysis, vascular bypass surgery, transplants, and other measures. However, these procedures cannot restore quality of life. Individuals who are on hemodialysis spend the majority of their time in dialysis centers or in hospitals getting their A-V shunts or grafts repaired constantly. These patients would not wish the pain and suffering associated with kidney dialysis on their worst enemies. I have yet to see a graphic visual TV documentary on the daily routine of a kidney patient or diabetic patient with serious vascular disease. At every step viewers should be made aware of the horrific nature of these self-inflicted problems that most patients endure.

In recent years, gastric bypass surgery has been heralded as the new miracle for people who are dangerously obese and cannot control their eating. Gastric bypass surgery makes the stomach smaller and allows food to bypass part of the small intestine. It forces people to eat less, and when they do eat, fewer calories are absorbed.

I have no doubt that this surgery has been a lifeline to many desperately obese people, but don't think that it's an easy solution. Gastric bypass is an extremely serious operation, with many dangerous side effects. More to the point, it will not solve your overeating problem if you haven't made a mental adjustment to eat healthfully. You may lose a great deal of weight in the first few years after the surgery, but if you still crave all the foods you once ate when you were obese, you will put on some weight. For example, I recall one patient who couldn't eat chocolate cake anymore who would sip chocolate syrup instead. Ten years after their surgery, 20 percent of gastric bypass patients have managed to regain their lost weight. This is a clear example of the fact that overeating is an emotional, not a physical, problem. We don't bypass the emotions, just the stomach. If we could perform an emotional bypass, there would be no need for a stomach bypass. Ignore the emotional component, and failure is inevitable.

No More Denial

I want everyone to think for a second about the consequences of overeating before the next doughnut or bagel smothered with cream cheese touches their lips. Only then do we have a chance to contain the overeating habit and its follies. I personally don't believe in doomsday predictions. But if there is a doomsday, the threat is certainly not coming from out of this world. It's coming from our inner selves—our insatiable drive to seek pleasure at any cost from food, drugs, sex, and material possessions. Arrogance, pleasure seeking, and the inability to be content are traits that have always plagued humans, but they are getting stronger in modern society. We no longer forage for food; it arrives on a silver platter. The more pleasure we derive from it, the more we crave. As a people, we have little memory of the simple contentment over a life well lived that our forefathers experienced. Today, we want more. We feel entitled to more. And it threatens to be our ruination.

Our forefathers definitely had healthier eating habits than us, and they also led more active but simpler lifestyles. They expected a lot less from life and were contented if most of their expectations were met. Today, we expect more in life and are easily disappointed. Such disappointments can drive a person to seek comfort in food, leading to unhealthy eating habits or overeating. We are not happier today than our forefathers. Nor are we healthier.

I realize that this is not a message people want to hear. It is

uncomfortable to be confronted with blatant excess and gluti-
nous cravings. We don't like to think of ourselves as grasping individuals. We claim to have a higher purpose. But actions speak
louder than words. And the truth lies in the undeniable epidemic of obesity.

3

A Problem of the Mind, Not the Body

"DR. PRASAD, I must have a death wish. I need your help." Maria, fifty-eight, spilled out her anxiety before I could even greet her. As I did not see a loaded gun in her hand, I told her that her situation could not be all that bad. I told her to take a deep breath and settle down in the chair and tell me why she felt so bad about herself. Maria relaxed enough to smile and then said, "I am my own worst enemy."

I asked her to explain what she meant by that.

"Sure," she said. "It's easy. My doctor tells me constantly that if I don't lose fifty pounds, I'll soon become a full-fledged diabetic. But I can't stop snacking on potato chips, sweets, candy, and cake. I binge, then get mad at myself, get depressed, and binge some more. Does that answer your question?"

Maria believed there was a kink in the hard wiring of her brain that made her overeat. But the compulsion to overeat is a problem of the *mind,* not of the brain. As any person enslaved by a bad habit will tell you, it is not enough to know intellectually that something is bad for you and should be stopped. Most of my patients are completely baffled by their inability to respond to the most persuasive arguments about the harm their behavior is causing to their health, relationships, careers, and well-being. The reason for this disconnection lies in the complex nature of the mind, which involves the dynamic interplay of three divisions—intellect, emotions, and instinct.

If you truly want to stop overeating for good, you must understand the way your mind is interfering with your resolve to change.

The Mind's Delicate Balance

This is the way your mind works. The Intellectual Division of the mind receives information then presents it to the Emotional Division for acceptance. The Emotional Division is the real policymaker, the one that calls the shots. When you can't break a habit it is because your mind's Intellectual Division has failed to make its case for giving up the habit to the Emotional Division, which says, Sorry, I'm not convinced. This behavior feels good to me. Without the support of the Emotional Division, both the Intellect, which executes proper actions to safeguard you, and the Instincts, which control your habitual behavior, are incapable of making short- or long-term corrections. The only argument strong enough to jar the Emotional Division into compliance would be a radical one, such as, The next doughnut you eat will kill you. This is not realistic, and therefore cannot be used as a convincing argument by the Intellect.

The human mind is a most effective, complex, and mysterious entity. It is capable of devising swift, savvy, and ingenious maneuvers to help us survive a harsh and ever-changing world. The mind, whose job it is to protect the interests of the individual, attempts to manipulate environmental forces to its advantage. When it fails to do so, it has no choice but to grudgingly adapt to the environmental requirements in order to survive. Unfortunately, when the environment and the mind do not see eye to eye, the mind suffers and the individual pays a heavy toll in health, happiness, and even survival. Obviously, the mind has an extremely difficult assignment, with little room for error. Let's examine the interplay among the three divisions to better grasp these complex dynamics.

THE INTELLECTUAL DIVISION

The Intellectual Division harbors the pragmatic component of the mind, which we know as human intelligence. The individual characteristics of this intelligence are reasoning, judgment, logic, discretion, calculation, imagination, analysis, and anticipation. By virtue of these segments, the Intellectual Division is also known as the rational division of the human mind. It is the most complex, sophisticated, and highly evolved section of the mind. Each and every component of the Intellectual Division exhibits a unique natural gift of its own, which comes in handy in fulfilling this division's responsibility to absorb and analyze the barrage of information it receives from the environment, and to program an appropriate response. It appears that nature has picked each and every one of these components for their distinct talent, and purposefully grouped them together under one banner. This ingenious assortment of incredible characteristics has boosted the Intellectual Division to the front lines of our struggle for survival.

Utilizing the services of our five senses—sight, smell, hearing, taste, and touch—the Intellectual Division receives a steady stream of divergent messages and information from the environment. The individual components of the Intellectual Division analyze millions of bits of information and prepare an appropriate response. If the input from the environment is processed in the Intellectual Division without any interference or influence from the Emotional Division, the outcome of its analysis would be uniform and universal for everyone. Thus, despite a diversified ethnic as well as geographic background, one would expect a stereotyped response to the environment from every human being of similar intellectual caliber. But in reality, this is not the case. No two human beings are alike. They do not think the same way or have the same interests. Different human beings see the same set of facts from unique perspectives. This diversity is caused primarily by the influence of the Emotional Division.

The Emotional Division

The Emotional Division, which I consider to be the most powerful conscious counterpart of the Intellectual Division, accommodates two sets of powerful emotions—primitive and advanced. Primitive emotions are anger, rage, pain, pleasure, comfort, thrill, fear, fright, and selfishness. These primitive emotions are shared by almost all larger mammals. Advanced emotions are love, caring, affection, passion, compassion, concern, grief, deceit, jealousy, hate, greed, pride, and prejudice. The advanced emotions are shared by animal species of a higher intellectual order. The type and the number of advanced emotions are determined by the level of intelligence of the animal species. Human beings are the sole possessors of all levels of emotions, but the primitive emotions often remain the most potent. Love, affection, compassion, and concern are very advanced and usually take a backseat to all others. They tend to lose out in an argument to more powerful, primitive emotions and to their close allies—jealousy, greed, hate, and vengeance. This fact is most evident in the human propensity to wage war.

All human beings are born with the same capacity for expressing emotions, but there is an individual variation in the intensity of the influence that each emotion has on the overall function of the mind. For example, in some people rage and anger may have a stronger influence than compassion and tolerance. Likewise, in others greed, jealousy, and selfishness may mute the influence of other advanced emotions. Therefore, the Emotional Division is the major deciding factor for the individual differences among human beings. This division is also responsible for the overall disposition, attitude, and outlook of a person. In fact, it is the Emotional Division that generates the necessary drive for all advanced life-forms (animals and humans) to initiate an action. Without emotions human beings would remain passive reactionaries. With emotions we are aggressive activists.

The Emotional Division of the human mind shapes our character and our response to the environment. Just imagine if human beings did not have emotions. We would be reduced to nature-created robots—expressionless, mechanical zombies programmed to survive. It is the Emotional Division, not the Intellectual Division, that most sets us apart from lower animals.

The Irrational Nature of Emotional Decision Making

For all practical purposes there is a barrier, like the Great Wall of China, separating the Intellectual Division from the Emotional

Division and the Instinctual Division. This barrier acts as a screening agent for the Emotional Division. Like any effective screener, it fully understands the Emotional Division's needs, requirements, and directives. It screens all incoming messages from the Intellectual Division and lets in only those that appeal to the emotions. This screening agent is nonexistent at birth and appears sometime during early childhood. In the beginning stages, it is a nonselective weak barrier. As a child grows, the barrier becomes stronger and more selective. By early or mid teens, it develops into a full-fledged selective barrier. This barrier is not passive. Its structural integrity is guarded by the Intellectual Division and its functional integrity is controlled by the Emotional Division. The Emotional Division dictates terms to the agent that fulfill its own needs. This arrangement leaves very little room for the Intellectual Division to force its messages through to either the Emotional Division or the Instinctual Division.

When the Emotional Division is in a state of distress or turmoil, it can block messages coming from the Intellectual Division. Rational thought is inhibited by the powerful emotional drives. No wonder when you lose your cool or composure, you cannot think or act straight. Only the Intellectual Division is capable of understanding the world we live in and assessing the situations we encounter. However, because it has only conditional access to the rest of the mind, it is forced to compute its response based on the input from the Emotional Division, which can be irrational.

This interplay has great relevance to productive habits, such as playing golf or performing surgery, as well as counterproductive habits, such as overeating. When the Intellectual Division concludes that continuing to overeat presents a threat to an individual's survival, it takes a Herculean effort to convince the Emotional Division to concur.

Many people who come to my office are disgusted and disenchanted by their inability to stop their compulsive eating. They know they're hurting themselves—I don't have to tell them. But their intellects are blocked from receiving these healthy messages by the intransigent Emotional Division, which compels them to continue overeating regardless of the consequences.

THE INSTINCTUAL DIVISION

The Instinctual Division is the unconscious counterpart of the Intellectual and Emotional Divisions. This division plays a crucial role in our struggle for survival as it holds the directives from nature. Nature expresses its intent through the Instinctual Division via three basic directives: (1) protection of self, (2) preservation of the surrounding environment to support the self, and (3) propagation of the self. These fundamental directives from nature are incorporated in our mind as basic instincts—thus the name Instinctual Division. However, in the case of humans, nature has expanded this division to accommodate countless useful acquired or learned habits. Here's the catch: only when the Intellect and the Emotions are in harmony can an individual recognize his talents and be able to polish them as tools of survival. Therefore, a pragmatic outlook and a healthy attitude are essential in the struggle for survival.

For lower animals, whose learning capacity is limited by meager intellect and a narrow range of emotions, learned behavior pales when compared to unlearned, primary instinctual behavior. Humans are the opposite. By virtue of a wide array of advanced emotions, primitive emotions, and a powerful and versatile intellect, learned behavior not only overshadows but also modifies unlearned primary behavior. With humans, the interpretation of nature's directives and the choice of acquired habits are largely up to the individual.

Lessons from the Wild

Diet and nutrition is a vast business in this country, but we could save a lot of money if we learned from animals in the wild. They've figured out how to eat right. Why can't we? Despite our advanced intelligence and the knowledge of modern science, we have yet to come up with a sensible formula for a healthy, balanced meal. We are still debating over the right mix of protein, carbohydrates, and fat. What do animals have that we lack when it comes to eating habits?

Animals in the wild rely mainly on their instincts for survival, while humans have shifted from our instincts to our emotions and intellect for our daily needs, safety, and security. When it comes to eating, which is a fundamental requirement for survival, animals have beaten us by letting their instincts guide them. In this instance, I believe their limited intellectual capacity and lack of advanced emotions may be a blessing in disguise. Over the years, we have slowly but surely let our emotions disengage the instincts from our eating habits. With their instincts intact, animals eat to live. With emotions in charge of our eating habits, we live to eat. Until we restore our instincts as the designers of our eating habits, all of the Food Pyramids, diet books, and nutritional experts in the world will not help us eat right.

When it comes to food, humans are constantly fighting against the development of healthy instincts. When a child is born, we immediately force the instincts to take a backseat by subjecting the child to a pediatrician's prescribed eating plan of formula/breast milk along with the number of times and how much a baby should be fed, instead of encouraging the baby to rely on its natural hunger instinct. Does the pediatrician know more than nature? A baby's natural hunger is sidelined from the first day. I have seen many parents who are so rigid in following feeding schedules, it doesn't matter whether the baby is sleeping or hungry. The baby has to be fed at the precise moment and the prescribed quantity of food. After only a few days in such an atmosphere, an infant will start demanding milk based on the time of day, not hunger. No wonder people are primed to eat by the time of the day, sight of food, smell of food, or the setting, rather than their hunger instinct. Animals eat when they are hungry and stop when their stomachs are full. They do not even bother to look at food until hunger strikes again, which could be hours or days. By munching the whole day, humans have totally disconnected the hunger instinct from our feeding habit. For animals, food is not a symbol of prestige, ambience, and fashion. Nor is it a pleasure-seeking device or a tool of courtship or camaraderie. For them food is a necessary tool of survival. Nature is the wisest and smartest teacher in the entire universe and teaches animals to eat right, through their instincts. Remember that nature conveys its rules and regulations to each of us, including animals, through our instincts. When we sideline the instincts, we are indirectly disregarding nature and its mandate.

In India, there is a popular book about how to survive in the jungle. It advises that when you aren't sure which substances are safe to eat, you should follow the monkeys. Eat leaves, fruits, or roots that monkeys eat, and avoid the foods that monkeys pass up. Otherwise, you may die of food poisoning. Somehow, monkeys know which fruit is safe to eat and which is poisonous. Where did the monkeys learn to distinguish one fruit from another? Such skills are innate to animals and are needed for their survival. Unfortunately, we humans have let our instincts lag behind our emotions and intellect rather than work with them as equal partners in the struggle for survival.

Another example is animals that live in the polar regions, like bears and penguins. These animals need lots of dietary fat as an effective deterrent against the cold weather, as well as a reservoir of nutrition for the harsh winters. Fat is an essential tool for survival as dictated by nature, and these animals have the biological makeup—enzyme systems, cardiovascular systems, livers, kidneys—designed to handle large quantities of fat. Scientists have long tried to figure out why animals in the polar regions are spared from obesity, heart disease, high blood pressure, and diabetes, given their fat intake. But the answer is obvious—their bodies need fat, but human bodies are not designed by nature to tolerate an excess amount.

Here is a case in point. In 2005, a twenty-three-year-old football player named Thomas Herrion died suddenly of a heart attack. How could this happen to a young athlete? Herrion's death was mainly attributed to his weight. He was considered obese, even for a football player. Since he was physically active, his large body mass took a toll on his vital organs. The medical examiner concluded that his heart could not tolerate the brunt of his body weight.

The average weight of a football player today is around three hundred pounds. That is 25 percent higher than a player in the 1980s. More than 56 percent of players are considered obese, and 26 percent are considered morbidly obese. Sports agents contend that if a player is below three hundred pounds, it's almost impossible to secure a contract from a football franchise. Why? Because their opponents are getting bigger, too.

Can you see the difference between a polar bear and a football player? Nature expects the bear to be fat to survive. Therefore, its cardiovascular system is designed to withstand the extra weight. However, a football player is not a bear. He is a human being. The basic blueprint of his vital organs is different.

To stop overeating for good, you must see your task as that of restoring the balance of the mind and reinstalling your natural instincts.

Emotional Eating:
The Mind Stages a Revolt

Joan is the office manager for a large insurance company, located on the eighth floor of a high-rise building. One day, the elevators in her building broke down, and at the end of business hours the employees had to take the stairs. Joan is obese, and she suffers from several related problems, the most troublesome being moderate to severe arthritis and neuritis. When the weather is hot and humid, she feels that her feet are literally on fire. The pain in her back, knees, and feet become unbearable if she walks and stays on her feet for even fifteen minutes.

When she learned that the elevators were down, Joan knew she had two choices: she would either have to walk down eight flights of stairs or camp out in her office. The rest of the office staff had already started to walk down the stairs, and Joan didn't want to embarrass herself by staying behind, so she followed her colleagues. After three flights, she began to feel excruciating pain in her knees. She rested for fifteen minutes before she proceeded down the remaining flights. By the time she reached the bus stop, which was an additional ten-minute walk, she had missed the bus. She had to wait another thirty minutes before the next bus came, and there was no place to sit at the bus stop. By the time the bus arrived, her feet were burning, and it was standing-room only. She suffered all the way home, and by the time she finally arrived, she was almost in tears. The sad feeling turned into anger, and in a state of rage she stormed out of her apartment, got into her car, and drove to the nearest pastry shop. She bought chocolate cake and cookies. Her resolve to diet hit the dust for that day. The next day when she awoke, she was upset and her whole body ached. She called in sick, stayed home, and ate more.

The next day, Joan returned to work, once again resolving to conquer her eating problem. Joan had spent her life yo-yoing between dieting and overeating, and diets never worked. During the short intervals she dieted, she felt a storm brewing inside her and exploded at the slightest provocation. However, her obesity had created real health consequences, and she feared that soon her arthritis would make her immobile.

Joan had managed to control her symptoms with the medication Celebrex. But when studies showed that Cox-2 inhibitors like Celebrex were linked to heart attacks, her doctor informed her that he was taking her off Celebrex for the time being, and recommending ibuprofen for relief from pain and inflammation.

Joan was very upset. She reminded her doctor that the reason she had originally started taking Celebrex was the fact that ibuprofen upset her stomach. She couldn't return to that misery. She pleaded with her doctor to keep her on Celebrex.

Joan's doctor felt that he was in a real bind. He could not in good conscience allow Joan to continue taking Celebrex, because her obesity and high blood pressure made her a prime candidate for heart attack. Frustrated by Joan's neglect of her own best interests, he snapped at her, saying, "If you'd lose some weight, we wouldn't have this problem."

Joan was crushed by his words. She needed understanding and support, not admonitions and ultimatums. At that moment, she felt that the whole world had turned against her. She drove straight from the doctor's office and consoled herself with forbidden foods.

Is there any question that Joan's eating behavior was triggered by emotional distress? The answer is an absolute no. If you are reading this book, you may identify with Joan's struggle, and her feelings of powerlessness. The good news is that knowing the problem is emotional means that help is not beyond your control.

4

The Myth of Appetite

HERE IS A RADICAL THOUGHT: appetite does not exist in the natural world. Nature installed a drive in all creatures as a cue to replenish depleted energy stores. That drive is called hunger. Appetite, however, is an invention of human emotions. When overeaters complain that they have trouble controlling their appetites, they are really describing an emotional need to seek pleasure or comfort in food, not a real hunger.

Our focus on appetite signals a total breakdown between the hunger drive and eating behavior. Who can deny that it is one of the leading causes of obesity?

To prove this point, I conducted a small experiment in the coffee lounge at the hospital. One day I arranged an enticing display of doughnuts, pastries, and bagels and cream cheese next to the coffeepot. Between 10:00 A.M. and noon, twenty-seven people came into the coffee room, and all but three of them helped themselves to food along with coffee. I asked each person who ate the following five questions:

1. Did you have breakfast this morning? If so, at what time?
2. Had you planned on eating anything more before lunch?
3. What time do you usually have lunch?
4. Are you still planning to eat lunch?
5. Were you hungry when you ate just now?

Here are the results:

Everyone had eaten breakfast before coming to work, and most were not planning to eat again until lunch. They came into the coffee room for a cup of coffee or to relax, and were not expecting to eat because they did not know that food was being served.

Most of the people who ate from the platter saw no connection between eating a snack and having lunch. They planned to have their usual midday meal.

When I asked the final question, I got some strange looks, which I interpreted as "Why should I have to be hungry to eat a doughnut?" Not one person acknowledged being hungry when they ate. They ate because it was there.

I was more curious about the three people who chose not to eat from the platter. They all said that they didn't eat snacks between meals. It's no surprise that none of the three was overweight.

Invariably, people who eat without thinking consume more food than those who pay attention to what they eat. These are the very ones who tell me that they have trouble controlling their appetites. But they are hard-pressed to describe the actual physical symptoms of appetite. I am certain this is because there are none.

The Diet Pill Fallacy

Appetite suppressants have long been the most popular form of weight control. Who doesn't love the idea of a magic pill that is capable of corralling one's great appetites? I have rarely met an overeater who has not tried appetite suppressants at some point. But in my opinion, appetite suppressants, which usually have amphetamine-like qualities, win the prize for the biggest failure in weight management. For one thing, they don't work since they are merely addressing a phantom condition. Worse still, the side effects of appetite suppressants can be dangerous and even deadly.

My patient Fran, who had been engaged in a losing battle with eating for most of her life, told me with a wistful nostalgia of her experience with appetite suppressants some years earlier. In high school a friend had introduced her to the amphetamine Dexedrine. "The few months I took those pills were the happiest of my life," she told me. "I felt so good, so energized. I didn't care about food. The weight melted off. It was magical. I finally felt like a normal human being. Boys looked at me, my friends complimented me. Until then, I'd never thought I could be pretty or sexy."

"If Dexedrine was so wonderful, why did you stop taking the pills?" I prodded, wanting to hear Fran's version of events.

Fran told me that the euphoria and disinterest in food lasted about four months. Then, gradually, she started feeling down and missing her favorite foods. She added an extra pill to her daily dosage, thinking it would help. After another week, she realized that although she had less desire to eat, she thought about food almost constantly. And she didn't feel the euphoria she had once felt. Instead, she was troubled by sleep disturbances and headaches.

Over a year's time, Fran continued to take Dexedrine, increasing the dosage a couple of times. She lost fifty pounds and looked great, but she felt lousy. The side effects of the drug were constant, including continued sleep problems, light-headedness, agitation, headaches, and slight tremors in her hands. These effects were compounded by nutritional deficiency, because Fran was barely eating enough to keep a bird alive.

Despite the side effects, Fran felt that taking Dexedrine was well worth it. Then she began to have nosebleeds. These worried her, but she shrugged them off, thinking that everyone got nosebleeds sometimes. One day at school she felt terribly dizzy. She thought her head was exploding into a thousand pieces and the world was closing in on her. She passed out, and when she regained consciousness, she was in the ER with an IV drip inserted in her hand. Her mother was hovering worriedly by her bedside.

"What happened?" she weakly asked her mother.

Fran learned that she'd fainted and started convulsing in the school hallway. A teacher called 911, and an ambulance took her to the hospital. When she arrived at the emergency room, her heart was beating very fast and the rhythm was irregular. At first, the doctors had no clue as to what had happened to her. Later, blood tests revealed toxic levels of amphetamines in conjunction with low proteins, low sodium, and low potassium. The ER doctors told her mother that Fran was lucky to be alive. When she returned from the hospital she knew that was the end of her tryst with the magic pills.

To understand what happened to Fran, we must understand

the insidious effects of an amphetamine like Dexedrine on the body's chemical balance. At first, the effects of the drug seemed positive to Fran, especially the euphoria and the sudden disinterest in food. However, from the outset, her body was preparing to launch a response to this foreign intruder. Until that time, approximately two months into her Dexedrine use, the drug had free access to Fran's nervous system. Her emotions were happy on two counts. First, her looks improved rapidly. Second, the altered chemical environment of the brain had suppressed the appetite center and she didn't feel as if she was making a sacrifice when she didn't eat. Her emotions did not register sacrifice. In other words, Fran did not feel deprived of not eating her favorite foods. But as her brain cells became resistant to the influence of the chemical agent, Fran started to crave her favorite foods again, which made her uneasy. By then she had lost a considerable amount of weight, so her resistance was low. Like many dieters, Fran thought that once she'd lost the weight, she could return to her previous eating habits without suffering any consequences. Naturally, this didn't happen. When she began to put on weight, she increased the dosage of the Dexedrine, which didn't produce the euphoria she'd felt before, but did affect her blood pressure and heart rate. The lack of proper nutrition exacerbated her condition, and she narrowly escaped death.

Given this frightening experience with Dexedrine, one would think that Fran would look back on those days with horror. Instead, she was wistful. She had never repeated the feeling of euphoria. Nor had she ever managed to suppress her appetite without great effort. She confessed to me that she wished scientists would come up with a safe form of Dexedrine—one that would permanently fill her with happiness and give her a lifetime of control over her eating.

"I regret to inform you that such a pill will never exist," I said. "Even if it did, is that what you really want? Wouldn't you prefer to get off this treadmill altogether?"

She had to think about it for a minute, but she finally agreed that she would.

"Good," I said. "In that case, I'll tell you a secret. Appetite doesn't exist, only hunger. There is no need for you to suppress a phantom. Only to learn how to recognize the real physical hunger signals."

Fran looked at me with tears in her eyes. In one statement I had broken through a lifetime of fear and helplessness. Now she was ready to get down to the real business of changing her eating habits and her life.

A WORD ABOUT EATING DISORDERS

I believe that life-threatening eating disorders, such as anorexia nervosa and bulimia, have their basis in complex emotional drives. However, this book is not for people who are pathologically afflicted in these ways. They need immediate hands-on help.

In the beginning, bingeing and purging may seem like a benign activity, practiced mostly by teenage girls to control their weight. But over time, the side effects of chronic bingeing and purging include a destruction of the esophageal tract, nutritional deficiency, stress on the heart and major organs, and collapse of the digestive system. Unfortunately, what begins as an easy way to stay slim can grow into a full-fledged crisis. When bulimics try to stop the cycle, they usually experience severe withdrawal symptoms typical of an addictive habit. These include agitation, depression, and sleep disturbances.

Although this book focuses on overeating, it is important to point out that *under*eating is the flip side of the coin. It is a manifestation of the same emotional drive that centers around food. Primary anorexia is a pathological mental disorder that is devastating to individuals and families. Since it mostly afflicts otherwise healthy young girls, it is a great shock to parents when they observe their daughters becoming skeletons before their eyes.

I have treated many people for anorexia. I believe the fundamental problem is a disconnection in the mind between food and its role in survival. There is no compulsion or desire to eat. Anorexics believe that eating less and less is the only way to feel good and secure. At the same time, they vehemently deny that it is an act of suicide. These girls are usually not depressed, but they are definitely defiant and disillusioned. They do their best to keep family and friends out of their affairs, and they resent it when their loved ones "side with food" against them.

We have much to learn about the powerful forces that drive young girls to obsessively binge and purge, or to starve themselves. If you or someone you love suffers from an eating disorder, it's important to get help from a professional trained in the emotional and physiological aspects of these syndromes. Don't delay. It could be a matter of life and death.

No Easy Road

My obese patients are always eager to get disciplined to lose weight, as if discipline were a commodity one could lease until the goal was accomplished. But discipline doesn't appear in bits and pieces whenever you need it. If you have discipline, you have it all the time. Either you have it or you don't. It is possible for you to develop discipline as a quality you will cherish for the rest of your life. An individual who exhibits discipline in one area can more easily extend it to other areas of life.

Martin, a federal judge in his mid-fifties, came to me for help losing about thirty-five pounds. During the initial consultation, as Martin told me about himself, I saw that he had come from humble beginnings and worked his way up to his highly respected position. He had exhibited a great deal of discipline to build a stable, satisfying life for himself and his beloved wife and children. I wondered why an individual of such high caliber, principles, and discipline was struggling so hard to keep his weight under control.

I asked Martin to explain in his own words why he had failed to keep his weight under control when he had done so well in other areas of his life. He was surprised by my question, but he realized the validity of it. After thinking it over for a couple of minutes, Martin said, "I really don't know. I can't come up with any explanation other than lack of willpower."

I think I knew what he meant by lack of willpower. The script went something like this: *I would like to lose weight, look good, and feel healthy, but I don't have the time or patience to endure the hard work involved in the process. I'd prefer to delegate the task of keeping my weight under control to someone else.*

With this understanding, I said to Martin, "Sir, willpower is always in short supply, and I have placed an order for several units to service my other patients. If you wish, I can place an order for you. As soon as the package arrives, I will ask you to come in and have it installed in your mind."

Martin laughed appreciatively. He got the message and decided to put his customary discipline to work on managing his weight. Two years later, Martin was in better shape than he'd been since he was young. I knew all along that he could do it if he made the commitment. Martin already had the needed discipline at his disposal. All he had to do was extend it in the direction of his eating habits.

In order to successfully stop overeating, you must be uncomfortable with your habit. Obviously, as long as you are comfortable, you have little motivation to change. But something converts the comfortable habit into the uncomfortable habit—health issues, family problems, professional or social interferences, spiritual issues, and so on. You must want to stop overeating. You can no longer bear the idea of continuing. You may try to give up the habit, but fail repeatedly. The desire to break the habit grows into a firm resolve or commitment to become permanently and happily free of it.

Part Two

The Prasad Method: Mind Over Habit

HUMAN BEINGS take actions based on what they *believe,* not what they *know.* Your knowledge of the facts may convince you that something has to be done to prevent a catastrophe, but that is not enough to compel you to act. Only when you believe that your life and well-being is hanging in the balance will you take action. Belief is centered in the Emotional Division of your mind, and true commitment emanates from your heart (emotions), not from your intellect. Once you are committed from the heart, you are certain to win your battle with overeating. You will no longer seek easy answers and quick fixes that sabotage your efforts. Instead, you will search for the truth about your condition and your options. Patience and perseverance will be your loyal companions.

Eating right is a lifelong occupation. It is not like giving up the smoking habit. You do not have to smoke to live, but you must eat healthfully to live and enjoy a satisfying life. Many of my patients consider this a bitter irony. The source of temptation is the very thing they need for survival. I invite you to change the way you view this dilemma. From now on, do not look at food and think "temptation." Look at food and think "nourishment." Love yourself and want what's best for you, and the rest will follow.

My program involves five steps to stop overeating for good:

Step 1: Understand why you must change your habit. Set aside superficial external motivations, and forge a lasting commitment from within that will stand the test of time.

Step 2: Identify your Overeating Profile. Discover the emotional triggers to your overeating, which are composed of six addictive drives: deprivation, entitlement, invincibility, disenchantment, insecurity, and defiance. Your Overeating Profile, which is formed by one or more of these drives, is the engine that charges up addictive behavior.

Step 3: Learn reality-based eating. Most dieters are easily persuaded by magical claims. It's time to accept the truth and discover how it will set you free.

Step 4: Make the change. Take the practical steps necessary to set yourself on the right course.

Step 5: Conquer the dieter's mentality. Bring closure to the eating habit that once consumed you, and move on to lead a life happily free of its constraints.

Are you ready to get started? Take a fresh notebook to help keep track of your journey or use the journal sheets in the Appendix of this book. Begin by stating your commitment in irrevocable terms. When questioned, people will often say, "I'd like to control my eating." This is not a commitment, only a wish. There is a big difference between wishful thinking and commitment. Wishful thinking leads people to give it a good try; when they fail, they will then say, "Better luck next time." When there is true commitment, failure is not an option.

Think of your commitment as a contract you are making with yourself that has no escape clause. To be successful, the contract must include:

- A decision to tackle the habit on its terms and conditions, not those you imagine or invent.
- A decision that failure is not an option.
- A decision to be not just free of the habit but *comfortable* and *productive* without the habit.
- A decision that you, not your habit, will decide your fate.

STEP 1

Understand Why You Must Change Your Habit

MAUREEN, a thirty-six-year-old nurse who weighed 193 pounds, told me that she wanted to lose at least fifty pounds. When I mentioned that she was embarking on a difficult task, she nodded and said she knew that, as she'd managed to lose a lot of weight a few years earlier through vigorous exercise and diet. Now that she'd gained it back, she was determined to try again. I asked her to tell me about her experience.

Six years ago, Maureen had fallen in love with Jerry, a lawyer who lived in her apartment complex. At the time, she weighed 189 pounds, and the romance took her by surprise. She had never imagined getting romantically involved at her weight, but once it happened, she was highly motivated to slim down. She wanted to be as attractive as possible for Jerry. She joined a health club and began a rigorous exercise program, along with a strict diet. As her weight dropped off, her romance progressed, and Maureen had never been happier.

Three years into the relationship, just when Maureen was expecting a marriage proposal, Jerry informed her that he'd met someone else. She was devastated. She cried for weeks, despairing of ever finding love again. And she ate—filling the emptiness in her heart with her old favorite foods. Within six months, she had regained her lost weight.

As I contemplated Maureen's sad story, I was once again struck by the insane phenomenon of intelligent human beings inflicting harm on themselves because someone else rejects them. It's an amazing thing that an external blow can lead us to do further harm to ourselves in a form of self-flogging.

Maureen was hurt by Jerry's infidelity and rejection, but instead of standing up to him and saying she didn't want a boyfriend who was so callous, she collapsed emotionally. I urged her not to let Jerry's cruelty destroy her peace of mind and weaken her resolve. I told her that we would embark upon a journey that was internal, not external. You see, Maureen's problem was her initial motivation for losing weight, which was to please the man she loved. When we change our habits to please another person, our efforts will eventually fail. Maureen needed to find her motivation from the inside out, not from the outside in.

The reasons why you want to stop overeating are as important if not more important than the reasons why you eat. You cannot be properly motivated for a lifetime of eating right if you are not serious about making an unconditional vow to yourself. Your commitment must come from the inside—not from the shallow desire to please a boyfriend or fit into a size 8 dress. External reasons will not stand the test of time.

Your commitment will stand the test of time if you have the right reasons—for example, self-respect and the desire to take care of your God-given body and mind.

Overeating is not an external reality, but an internal one,

which must be viewed from the inside out. Unless you fully understand yourself and your motivations, you have no hope of permanently releasing yourself from the habit. If you've tried to stop overeating before, only to fail, this time you'll start from an entirely different place. Instead of trying to wrestle the chocolate cake to the ground and demolish it, begin by trying to shift the focus from food to yourself. You are a unique individual. Your temperament, outlook, attitude, priorities, expectations, and limi-

THE RIGHT WAY: THE INSIDE-OUT APPROACH	THE WRONG WAY: THE OUTSIDE-IN APPROACH
Don't talk. Commit yourself.	Keep talking about going on a diet.
Plan your regimen carefully, relying on sound nutritional information and an understanding of your own compulsions.	Try the latest fad diet you see featured on TV.
Believe that overeating is unhealthy for your body, mind, and spirit.	Try to lose weight, but assume that if you fail, medical technology will rescue you.
Stop overeating for yourself—to improve your quality of life.	Lose weight to attract a mate or win the approval of others.
Rely on your patience, tolerance, and strength to defeat the discomfort.	Rely on diet pills or food replacements.
Concentrate on restoring your health.	Focus on being able to wear a desirable clothes size.
Make it your goal to become a healthy, happy eater for life.	Think of your diet as a "fix," and look forward to the day you can "go off" the diet.

tations are different from every other overeater. For this reason, only *you* can break your habit. Not your doctor, not a pill, not your husband, or therapist, or support group. Just you.

The hardships you are encountering are mainly due to your own choices. You're responsible for your predicament, and you must spearhead the campaign to save yourself. This job cannot be delegated. So stop looking outside yourself and relying on the judgment of others. This task belongs to you. Write your internal reasons for making this major change in your journal, and refer to them often.

STEP 2

Identify Your Overeating Profile

TO BE EFFECTIVE against your overeating, you must focus on the invisible enemy—the internally generated drives that feed it. By fixating on the external features, you may control your eating for a short time, but you will never get rid of the compulsion to overeat. As long as the compulsion is alive, you will eventually return to your prior behavior.

The key to your habit is the underlying drives that comprise your Overeating Profile. These drives are always lurking in the background of the habit. The stress of these drives primes the craving to eat. Think of the mind of an overeater as an emotional pressure cooker, fed by one or more elements of the Overeating Profile. As the pressure builds, you experience a growing discomfort, exhibited by agitation, rage, sleeplessness, the inability to concentrate, and so on. Most of my patients say they feel a battle going on in their minds, a void in the pit of their stomachs, and a preoccupation with food. The stress builds. At some point, when the psychological pressure becomes unbearable, the desire to eat turns into a ravaging craving to release the pressure.

These intense cravings are caused by an emotional need, not by actual hunger. That need comes from deeply rooted stories about why you need to eat to feel okay. The emotional drive of these stories allows you to continue behaviors that your rational mind clearly acknowledges as destructive. These drives are all-consuming. Often a person will have more than one of them. They trigger the Emotional Division to seek relief.

I totally reject the idea that the compulsion to overeat is driven by a chemical imbalance, food allergies, or any other physical basis. You are driven mentally to enjoy the attractive, beneficial experience from your eating habit. The overwhelming urge you feel to eat recklessly is strictly mental, not physical. That's why, even when you have short-term success on a diet, you eventually return to your old ways, driven by the overwhelming sense of deprivation, entitlement, invincibility, disenchantment, insecurity, and defiance that gave rise to the behavior in the first place.

None of us are completely free of these drives. They are integral to human emotions, and in a proper balance can even enhance our lives and motivate us to achieve. However, for people who exhibit addictive behavior, one or more of these drives take on a pathological character. For example, the normal influence of the Insecurity Drive is necessary to keep you alert and vigilant, thus enabling your survival. An overactive Insecurity Drive paralyzes you and impairs your ability to make decisions. It also fosters dependency by encouraging you to rely on an external crutch to get you through the day.

The Overeating Profile, which is formed by an imbalance in one or more of these drives, is the engine that charges up your self-destructive behavior. In this section, we will examine the drives of the Overeating Profile more closely, showing how an imbalance of one or more drives helps to keep you addicted. Take the quiz that is provided for each drive to determine whether it is out of balance for you. The results of these quizzes will provide essential clues to your overeating habit.

The Deprivation Drive

A healthy fear of deprivation is necessary for survival. It is the quality that has propelled humans to the top of the food chain. But when the struggle is no longer solely for survival, the Deprivation Drive occurs in the emotional division of the mind. The overeater consumes a certain amount of daily food for survival, but there is a point where the fear of feeling empty takes over.

Helen, a patient who came to me for help getting control over her compulsive eating, described her daily pattern like this: each day she started out trying to eat controlled portions of food in a balanced way, determined to listen to her hunger cues. When she got up in the morning, she ate a small bowl of whole-grain cereal with sliced fresh fruit and a glass of skim milk. At midmorning, she ate a small snack—an energy bar or a container of yogurt. So far, so good. But as the day progressed, Helen began to feel ravenous. Her hunger felt absolutely real. Her willpower was weakened. By lunchtime, she was consumed with thoughts of food. She'd make a beeline for a fast-food place, where she gulped down a large hamburger, French fries, and a thick milk shake.

Afterward, Helen always felt lousy. Her stomach was bloated and she felt sluggish and weak. Worse still, overeating led to more overeating. As she explained to me, "Once I fall off the wagon for the day, I'm a goner."

During the evening, alone and miserable in her apartment, Helen turned to food for solace. She soothed her misery with pasta and sauce, ice cream, and salty snacks. She called these her comfort foods, but they did not really provide comfort.

I asked Helen to describe what her cravings felt like. "Do you feel hungry?"

"No, not really," she admitted. Then she blurted out, "It's more like a feeling of sadness."

Inadvertently, Helen had identified the core of her problem. I complimented her on her honesty, and then asked, "When you overeat rich fattening foods, do you feel less sad?"

Helen bowed her head and there were tears in her eyes. "No. I feel worse. My stomach is full, but my heart is empty."

Once Helen acknowledged the emotional deprivation that drove her to overeat, it was the first step in a journey that would eventually reap positive results.

Many of the current treatments help overeaters focus on filling up that emptiness—with food replacements, medications, or appetite suppressants. They don't look at the individual and ask why you are compelled to overeat. Instead, they try to pacify your fear. None of these substitutes work for long, because the overeater still has the need to be pacified. You still feel deprived.

Is your Deprivation Drive out of balance? Take the following quiz to determine whether it plays a significant role in your eating behavior.

QUIZ: YOUR DEPRIVATION QUOTIENT

Read the following statements. In the box, give yourself
1 point for each statement that you agree with,
and 0 if it doesn't describe you.

STATEMENT	VALUE
You often feel physically tired or "burned out," especially toward the end of the day.	
On holidays and special occasions, your attitude is "Eat first, diet later."	
You frequently snack in between meals.	
You get up in the middle of the night to snack.	
You often feel lonely and wish you had more friends.	
You are easily overwhelmed by ordinary challenges, such as a crying child, a failed recipe, or a traffic jam.	
You think others have more opportunities or are luckier than you.	
Even when you're not planning to eat, the sight and smell of food compel you to eat.	

(continued)

You wish you had a spouse who could better understand your needs.	
You have a low tolerance for emotional discomfort.	

Score: Total the numbers in the right-hand column. That is your deprivation quotient. If your score is 1–5, you have a relatively normal Deprivation Drive. If your score is more than 5, your Deprivation Drive is overactive, making it a factor in your overeating.

The Entitlement Drive

A balanced sense of entitlement is important to your self-esteem. It allows you to feel special and motivates you to take care of yourself because your life is worth something. However, entitlement does not exist in the physical world. Nature does not play favorites. It does not give you a break because you work hard, or you're a nice person, or you're a genius. It does not care about your problems. Its terms and conditions are clear: behaviors have consequences. Just because you think you're entitled to reduce stress by snacking on fatty, high-calorie foods doesn't mean you'll avoid the many dire consequences associated with the habit. If your Entitlement Drive is overactive, you ignore nature's rules.

There is great power in acknowledging your place in the world, but many people cannot see this when they are obsessed with what others think and are only interested in imitating others because it feels good. Their reasoning is: everyone else feels entitled to a reward for their efforts, so why shouldn't I have one, too? Unfortunately, it is folly to follow the trend set by others without acknowledging the price tag of the reward.

Sam was a fifty-one-year-old corporate executive who marched into my office and announced, "I need to lose fifteen pounds."

I was somewhat annoyed. Sam gave the impression that he expected me to do it for him. Besides, to pay my fee for such a minor problem seemed like overkill.

"Save your money," I suggested. "You don't need me. Just cut down your food intake a bit and start walking. You'll lose the weight in no time."

Sam frowned, and then his face softened. "Look, if my problem was that simple, I wouldn't be here."

"Very well," I said, motioning to a seat. "Tell me about it."

Sam said that until he hit age forty-five he had never had to worry about his weight. Then the pounds started creeping up on him. In the past year he had put on more weight than in the previous four years, and the rate of weight gain alarmed him more than the actual number of pounds. At the same time he was furious that all of his extra weight had settled around his midsection. He felt that having a potbelly created a negative impression in business, and it certainly harmed his sex appeal.

Sam wasn't overly indulgent. He didn't eat junk food, rarely snacked, and wasn't that interested in sweets. But he disliked vegetables and considered himself "a real meat-and-potatoes man." A typical dinner would be a large steak, a baked potato with sour cream or butter, and half a bottle of red wine. He derived immense pleasure from this routine.

When I suggested to Sam that he consider replacing his steak with chicken or fish two or three times a week and start eating a salad or green vegetable instead of a baked potato, he exploded.

"That's just the response I expected," he said angrily. "Here I am, a reasonably fit guy. I don't smoke. I don't drink too much.

I don't fill up on junk. The one thing I get enjoyment from is meat, and now you want to take it away. I think I'm entitled to some pleasure in life."

I waited until he had said his piece and calmed down, then said, "You're wrong about one thing, Sam. I don't want to take away your steak. It's not mine to take away. In fact, I don't care if you eat steak three times a day."

"You don't?" He looked shocked.

"I don't make the rules," I said. "Nature does. And it seems that nature is saying that you have a choice: live with a potbelly or change your diet. You want a third choice, but it doesn't exist."

Sam's strong sense of entitlement made it difficult for him to accept nature's rules, but my straight talk reached him. In order to be successful, he realized he would have to let go of his attitude that he deserved a dietary reward. He gradually began to incorporate healthier foods into his diet, and began an exercise program.

Is your Entitlement Drive out of balance? Take the following quiz to determine whether it plays a significant role in your eating behavior.

QUIZ: YOUR ENTITLEMENT QUOTIENT

Read the following statements. In the box, give yourself
1 point for each statement that you agree with,
and 0 if it doesn't describe you.

STATEMENT	VALUE
You wish that you could eat as much as your friend eats and stay slim like her.	

You feel entitled to kick back and take a break every so often.	
You think you're justified in not always following the rules.	
"No pain, no gain" makes sense in theory but you don't think it applies to you.	
You believe that hard work and accomplishment should be rewarded in a tangible way.	
You tend to seek instant gratification.	
You consider yourself special.	
When you see something you want, you buy it.	
You believe in getting more for less.	
You often feel as if you deserve more.	

Score: Total the numbers in the right-hand column. That is your entitlement quotient. If your score is 1–5, you have a relatively normal Entitlement Drive. If your score is more than 5, your Entitlement Drive is overactive, making it a factor in your overeating.

The Invincibility Drive

No human being is invincible, but this drive can have a limited positive effect. It's the underlying sense of personal power that gives us courage in seemingly impossible situations. Out of balance, however, the Invincibility Drive is pure arrogance. It will stop you dead in your tracks. You are not God. You are not omnipotent. Overeaters with a strong Invincibility Drive don't really think their eating habits will eventually make them sick.

Sal, a fifty-seven-year-old restaurant owner, came to see me about his eating habits. He'd suffered a mild heart attack about three years earlier, and ever since had attempted to control his runaway eating habit. Unfortunately for Sal, his profession was his biggest obstacle. He owned three very successful Italian restaurants. He loved to cook, and he loved to eat.

Sal employed about one hundred people, including five chefs. He worked sixteen hours a day, in a high-stress environment, and was always surrounded by food. To relax, he loved nothing more than sitting down to a fine meal and a bottle of wine with his favorite customers, many of whom he'd known for years.

Immediately after his heart attack, Sal did lose some weight at the behest of his doctors and family. But a few months later he gained it back. He'd avoided the scale for six months and had skipped two appointments for stress testing. On some level, he thought he could avoid failure if he didn't face reality. His cardiologist was furious with him and threatened to drop him as a patient if he didn't clean up his act.

"I'm an old dog, but maybe you can teach me some new tricks," Sal suggested to me with a charming smile.

"Sorry, my bag of tricks is empty," I replied. "I just have reality."

Sal grimaced. I noticed a sense of arrogance in him. Even though he'd suffered a minor heart attack, the potential of another, more severe attack had not penetrated his psyche. As an entrepreneur and businessman, Sal was used to taking risks, and he thought that he could bargain with nature. But nature was an insurmountable foe. He would never win by going up against nature. He would have to learn to work with it.

Sal didn't like my message, but he reluctantly concurred with me. He really thought that by taking a few pills, like Lipitor for his cholesterol and aspirin to prevent blood clots, he could beat another heart attack. In the end, he realized that he would have to change his beloved routine.

We made an agreement that he would not eat or drink on the job. When he was hungry, he would go home, which was close by, and eat only his wife's cooking. He would restrict his alcohol intake to one or two glasses of wine a day, which he would drink only outside of his work environment. He also agreed that, with his cardiologist's approval, he would begin walking and build his stamina to the point where he could walk the mile and a half to and from work every day.

These lifestyle changes worked well for Sal, but he never could have implemented them if he didn't accept the fact that he wasn't invincible.

Is your Invincibility Drive out of balance? Take the following quiz to determine whether it plays a significant role in your eating behavior.

QUIZ: YOUR INVINCIBILITY QUOTIENT

Read the following statements. In the box, give yourself
1 point for each statement that you agree with,
and 0 if it doesn't describe you.

STATEMENT	VALUE
So far, you've experienced no real health problems from overeating, or if you have, you've minimized them.	

(continued)

You think there are exceptions to the rule, such as obese nonexercisers who live to be one hundred.	
You think of yourself as exceptionally strong.	
You like to beat the odds—in sports and at work.	
You are an eternal optimist.	
You march to your own drummer.	
You suffer from "tomorrow" syndrome. Every evening you plan to diet and exercise the next day, but the next day never comes.	
You are highly successful in your profession.	
You like to take risks.	
You have other addictive habits—such as smoking or gambling.	

Score: Total the numbers in the right-hand column. That is your invincibility quotient. If your score is 1–5, you have a relatively normal Invincibility Drive. If your score is more than 5, your Invincibility Drive is overactive, making it a factor in your overeating.

The Disenchantment Drive

Disenchantment is a necessary part of being human. We all have disappointments in life, and if we keep them in perspective we can learn from them. Out of balance, however, disenchantment can spiral into a sense of overwhelming gloom—the feeling that life has robbed you of joy. The wider the disparity between your expectations and the actual reality, the deeper the disenchantment. Many people who are diagnosed as clinically depressed are actually experiencing disenchantment. The Disenchantment Drive can play a role in overeating when depression triggers a heavy reliance on a crutch just to see you through the day.

Carol, forty-four, told me that she had always been a little chubby and had struggled to keep her weight under control. In the last four years, she had lost the battle, gaining more than forty pounds. The weight gain began shortly after her husband of twenty-three years died of cancer. She was unable to overcome her grief that he had died so young, cheating her of her soul mate when she had so many years to live. She was unable to help her two teenage daughters deal with their grief. Instead, they took on the role of her caretakers. She'd become a recluse, rarely going out. She stayed at home and ate to numb herself from her misery. As she started to put on weight, Carol, who had always been extremely careful of her appearance, figured it didn't make any difference. When her doctor warned her of the health consequences of her lifestyle, she shrugged and said to him, "Pete was a healthy guy, and he got cancer and died. It's a crapshoot."

Her doctor was concerned enough about Carol's state that he prescribed an antidepressant. The medication lifted her mood slightly, but it had no effect on her weight. Contrary to what many people believe, antidepressants are not helpful in weight control, as one of their side effects is weight gain. So, even as Carol was struggling to pull herself out of her depression, she continued to put on weight. A friend recommended that she see me, and now she was sitting in my office. What could I do for Carol?

Although Carol's purported reason for coming to me was for help losing weight, it was obvious that dieting was not the real solution to her problem. Until she came to terms with her emotions, I knew she would not win this battle. She used food as a consolation and to calm her nerves. She needed to disconnect food from her emotions if she wanted to eat right.

As we talked, Carol mentioned several times how much she loved her daughters. I decided to use this love as a tool to straighten up her emotions. I looked at her and asked, "Are you ready to face the truth? If not, I cannot help you."

"Dr. Prasad, I am willing to do anything to bring sanity into my life," she replied.

"Good. Then I must tell you, for an educated and loving person, you are really quite selfish."

Carol was shocked by my comment. She wasn't used to being challenged in this way. She demanded to know what I was talking about.

"Your household is in crisis," I said. "Instead of handling the situation wisely, you've turned into an emotional cripple. You care only about your own pain and disillusionment, not your children's welfare."

"It's just so unfair," Carol cried, tears spilling out of her eyes.

"Maybe so," I agreed. "But nature is not interested in your complaints. You cannot sit in your house and eat yourself sick, waiting for someone to come along and even the score for you."

At first, Carol thought I was cold and unsympathetic. But people who suffer from disenchantment don't need sympathy; they need a challenge. I'm certain that Carol initially agreed to work with me because she wanted to prove me wrong. Instead, she proved herself wrong. Her life wasn't over, after all. One year later, her daughters had their mother back. Carol ultimately chose not to be ruled by her disenchantment, and only then was she able to begin losing weight.

Is your Disenchantment Drive out of balance? Take the following quiz to determine whether it plays a significant role in your eating behavior.

QUIZ: YOUR DISENCHANTMENT QUOTIENT

Read the following statements. In the box, give yourself 1 point for each statement that you agree with, and 0 if it doesn't describe you.

STATEMENT	VALUE
You have not had the life you dreamed.	
You consider yourself a romantic.	
You wish you did not have a stressful job.	
You spend a lot of time in solitary pursuits.	
The only high point at work is your lunch break, when you can sit with others and relax for a few minutes.	
You often drink to excess or use recreational drugs to give yourself an edge and help you feel good.	
You believe that you are born to be fat and will stay fat for the rest of your life.	

(continued)

You tend to believe what will be will be.	
You have been treated for depression.	
You wish that your body could burn more calories than it is currently burning.	

Score: Total the numbers in the right-hand column. That is your disenchantment quotient. If your score is 1–5, you have a relatively normal Disenchantment Drive. If your score is more than 5, your Disenchantment Drive is overactive, making it a factor in your overeating.

The Insecurity Drive

The Insecurity Drive is the opposite of the Invincibility Drive. In proper balance these two drives give you a realistic idea of your potential. Out of balance, the Insecurity Drive involves a lack of courage to face the uncertain future, and a lack of confidence in your ability to tackle the challenges of a harsh world. Individuals with this drive hesitate to take action because they cannot be assured of the result. They forget that no human being has certainty about the future. They expect absolute reassurance that everything will work out fine. In the absence of this, they fret endlessly over minor issues. They are not proactive; they only know how to react. They long for peace of mind, but they never find it. Instead, they end up agitated and anxious.

In this quest to seek relief from their plight, they turn to substances that will numb their anxieties. We've all witnessed individuals binge on food, or gulp down alcohol, saying they do it to calm their nerves. Yet they are the most nervous people we know!

I believe that an underlying characteristic of the Insecurity

Drive is an extreme fear of rejection. To some extent all humans have a fear of rejection, because we are social beings. A healthy fear of rejection is actually a positive thing. It compels us to stay away from those who might hurt us. But people who are driven by this fear are extremely sensitive. They avoid getting close to others because they expect rejection. For them, overeating and obesity become a safe asylum.

Julie, thirty, was the only child of a dominant, overprotective, highly critical mother and a soft-spoken, mostly absent salesman father. When she came to my office, wanting to lose sixty pounds, I immediately saw that she was extremely sensitive and proud. She was also something of a loner who worked at home as a Web site designer. The Web is an ideal hideout for people who are insecure. Sight unseen, you can invent yourself freely. Julie admitted that she spent a lot of time on the Web in chat rooms, but she prayed for a normal relationship with a man.

When I asked Julie why she did not actively seek a relationship, she blushed. "Look at me," she said. "No man is going to be interested in me."

"Have you walked down the street lately?" I asked. "There are many men who are with larger women. That's an excuse. It isn't your weight that is preventing a relationship. But if you believe that being overweight prevents relationships, is it possible that you gained the weight to avoid them?"

Julie burst into tears at my words. I had struck a nerve. Her weight protected her from intimacy, which she was certain would lead to rejection. She would be unable to lose weight until she could face the world with courage and dignity.

Is your Insecurity Drive out of balance? Take the following quiz to determine whether it plays a significant role in your eating behavior.

QUIZ: YOUR INSECURITY QUOTIENT

Read the following statements. In the box, give yourself
1 point for each statement that you agree with,
and 0 if it doesn't describe you.

STATEMENT	VALUE
You experience disturbed sleep.	
You are nervous and filled with anxiety in social settings.	
You worry that others watch you and judge you lacking.	
You tend to be a pessimist.	
You consider yourself less attractive and less stylish than others.	
You grew up in an environment where adults were overly critical or overly protective of you.	
You are easily influenced to eat by others.	
You are eager to try every new fad diet without considering whether or not it is right for you.	
You wish you had a spouse or friend who would constantly encourage you to work out and eat right.	
You tend to eat more when you are sad and dejected.	

Score: Total the numbers in the right-hand column. That is your insecurity quotient. If your score is 1–5, you have a relatively normal Insecurity Drive. If your score is more than 5, your Insecurity Drive is overactive, making it a factor in your overeating.

The Defiant Drive

We all need a little defiance in our lives. It's what distinguishes us from robots. However, defiance for its own sake can get us into trouble. Many times an overeater continues the behavior as a gesture of defiance. The zeal of this drive is such that the overeater doesn't even worry about the consequences of his behavior or his own quality of life. He consistently downplays the risks or outright ignores them. In most cases the Defiant Drive is fueled by the Invincibility Drive.

Pam, forty, came to my office after repeated efforts to control her overeating ended in failure. She told me that women in her family tended to be overweight, and she had always been rigorous about keeping herself in shape.

"As you can see," she said, "I haven't been so rigorous in the last couple of years." Pam was far from obese, but she was carrying an extra twenty pounds on her small frame.

"What happened to change the discipline of a lifetime?" I asked.

"Oh, I don't know," she said with a sigh. "Things have just gotten away from me."

I asked her to tell me about her life, and we would see if there were clues that would provide an answer. Pam was an only child whose father owned a good business. When she was thirty, Pam met Craig, a sharp marketing executive with a major corporation. Soon after they were married, ill health forced Pam's father to turn the day-to-day running of the business over to Pam and Craig. They worked hard and the business grew. When Pam was thirty-five, she gave birth to twins, and stopped working to be home with them. They were starting kindergarten that year, and Pam was feeling restless. She missed working, and especially missed the sense of partnership she had felt when she and Craig were running the business together.

"So, why don't you go back to work with your husband?" I asked.

Pam's face clouded. Seeing that I had touched a nerve, I prodded a bit and learned that Pam was very resentful of her husband. She was sick of listening to him brag about how he had taken over her father's crumbling business and completely turned it around. Pam cringed at the insult to her father's hard work, and Craig's dismissal of her own contribution to the company. His boasting was a daily irritant that angered and depressed her, but she kept silent, not knowing how to articulate her feelings.

I was beginning to understand. "Tell me," I asked, "has your husband commented on your weight gain?"

"Only every day," she said. "He hates the way I've let myself go."

I realized that Pam's weight gain was an act of defiance—one that she wasn't fully aware of. It was a way she could exert power in a relationship where she felt diminished. Through her weight gain, which dismayed her husband, she could express her feelings of resentment.

When I shared this observation with Pam, she gaped at me. She truly hadn't realized what she was doing, but my words had the ring of truth.

"Talk to Craig," I suggested. "Get this off your chest. Then come back to me and we'll work on your overeating."

I believed that once Pam resolved her defiance, it would be easy for her to change her eating habits, as she had previously been quite disciplined. I was right. Craig agreed to go to couples therapy, and as their marriage improved, Pam's eating problem resolved itself. She never came back to my office, but called to say that she would have no trouble losing weight on her own.

Is your Defiant Drive out of balance? Take the following quiz to determine whether it plays a significant role in your eating behavior.

QUIZ: YOUR DEFIANCE QUOTIENT

Read the following statements. In the box, give yourself
1 point for each statement that you agree with,
and 0 if it doesn't describe you.

STATEMENT	VALUE
You have a short temper.	
You believe you were born to change the world for the better, and you believe you can.	
Other people don't understand your good motives.	
You eat more when you feel betrayed.	
Many people you come across are hypocrites.	
Powerful people don't care about the little guy.	
You consider food like truffles and caviar status symbols.	
You believe that sometimes the end justifies the means.	

(continued)

You've always had a troubled relationship with your parents.	
You believe that some people are born with slim and fit bodies and will stay that way even though they do not pay attention to what they eat.	
Score: Total the numbers in the right-hand column. If your score is 1–5, you have a relatively normal Defiant Drive. If your score is more than 5, your Defiant Drive is overactive, making it a factor in your overeating.	

Your Overeating Profile Score

Review your scores for each of the six drives, and make a note of where your score is more than 5. Write down in your journal the drive or drives you struggle with the most. This will be relevant to your later work.

If you are able, try to also write down the way the drive or drives manifest themselves in your life.

STEP 3

Learn Reality-Based Eating

OVEREATERS ARE USED TO being fed tall tales and swallowing them whole. The diet industry mostly sells products that don't work, yet the dieting population is always ready and willing to believe that the next diet program will be "the one." I don't know any other industry that could get away with such consistent failure and still have so many true believers. Usually, if a product doesn't work, people face reality and reject it. They don't keep going back, thinking, It didn't work yesterday, but maybe today will be different.

Most of my patients who struggle with eating and weight issues want to believe that their problems are the result of mysterious chemical interactions of which they haven't been apprised. When they ask, "What is the secret to controlling my weight?" they are disappointed in my reply: "There is no secret. It's very simple. Expend more calories than you consume."

"Oh, it couldn't be!" they cry. "What about my metabolism? What about my genes?" Yes, it's true that people are biological individuals. But I have yet to see a healthy person who follows the basic rules of nutrition gain excess weight.

A big part of changing the destructive emotional hold of eating is to face up to this truth. My program is reality-based. And let me tell you, once you accept reality, you'll never go back to fantasy. That's why the third step in my program is educating you to the truth about your body and the food you eat.

KNOW THE ENERGY DYNAMICS OF YOUR BODY

Once calories pass through your lips, you have no control over how your body handles them. Your body's natural mechanics set in motion their disposal and determines whether they are used for immediate energy or stored as fat for future needs. Your body will not waste valuable calories. If you choose to lose weight, you must operate within the parameters of the laws of nature. You must be smart to manage your energy equation for the rest of your life. If you handle this equation properly, eating right and maintaining proper weight is not difficult. Of course, overeating and gaining weight is a lot easier than eating right. But losing weight that you have gained is very difficult and maintaining the lost weight forever is even more difficult.

KNOW YOUR METABOLISM

Your basal metabolic rate (BMR) is the rate at which you burn calories. This is not a static number; it fluctuates as often as we blink our eyes because it is tied to activity.

BMR also varies among individuals. There are many factors that determine variations in BMR, including changes in daily activity, medical conditions, and genetics. I caution you to avoid using these variations as excuses to remain obese. Let's examine the variations and what they mean.

Genetic predisposition

For unknown reasons, some individuals are born with higher BMRs than others. However, these rates seem to make little difference in the ultimate potential for obesity. For example, Asians tend to have lower birth BMRs than Caucasians or African-Americans. However, as a group Asians are less likely to be obese. The differential is in the diet.

Age

The BMR of a newborn is relatively low, but reaches its maximum at the age of six or seven. After age eight, it takes a gradual slide downhill. At certain points of our lives, the downward slide becomes steeper. For example, adding new tissue requires more calories than replacing worn tissue, so there is a precipitous drop in BMR when our bodies stop growing at age twenty to twenty-four. There is a rise in BMR during pregnancy and lactation, but the rule of thumb is that BMR declines by one percent a year after age twenty-five.

Sex

Women typically have a lower BMR than men, and the rate of decline is faster than in men.

Hormones

Among all the body's hormones, our thyroid hormone has the maximum influence on BMR. It is well known that BMR is low in people with hypothyroidism (sluggish thyroid activity). Unfortunately, many desperate obese people are persuaded that their problems can be solved with thyroid hormones, which will boost their BMR and help them lose weight faster. It doesn't work that way. Thyroid hormone supplementation may relieve symptoms for people who truly have low thyroid function. But it does not seem to have any effect on BMR.

Climate

Warmer temperatures may slightly lower BMR, but it is when the weather turns cold that most people have trouble with weight gain. Winter blues and lack of exercise have more of an impact that natural climate changes.

Body surface area

People with smaller frames tend to have higher BMRs than larger individuals. Scientifically, body surface area is calculated in square meters. To determine your body surface area, multiply your height in centimeters by your weight in kilograms, and divide the result by 10,000.

Nutritional state

BMR is lower in malnourished people, which is why extreme starvation diets lead to sluggish metabolism.

Disease

Infection or fever boosts BMR by 12 percent for every one-degree increase.

Muscle/fat (M/F) ratio

There is a direct correlation between M/F ratio and BMR. The higher the M/F ratio—that is, the more muscle mass compared to fat—the higher the BMR. Regular physical exercise and healthy eating boosts the BMR by increasing muscle mass. The quality of muscle also has an effect on BMR. For example, a person with strong, firm muscles has a higher BMR than a person with flabby muscles, even though the M/F ratio may be the same. The M/F ratio is also slightly higher in men.

It is impossible to get a precise measurement of how many calories you utilize in a given day. But you can get a rough estimate, which will help guide you in establishing your eating and exercise plan.

CALCULATE YOUR BMR

The following calculations, one for men and one for women, establishes your resting BMR. That means roughly how many calories you burn every day just to be alive in a tranquil state. The average, moderately active person, burns about 30 percent more calories than the resting BMR.

Men
This calculation is for an average adult male, based on .9 calories per kilogram of weight per hour.

Example: 170-pound male
(Results are rounded off)

1. Convert pounds to kilograms (divide by 2.2):   77
2. Multiply by .9 for number of calories per hour: 69
3. Multiply by 24 for number of calories per day
   burned at rest: 1,656
4. Multiply by .30 and add the result: 2,153

This is your average calorie recommendations per day.

Women
This calculation is for an average adult female, based on .8 calories per kilogram of weight per hour.

Example: 145-pound female
(Results are rounded off)

1. Convert pounds to kilograms (divide by 2.2):   66
2. Multiply by .8 for number of calories per hour: 53
3. Multiply by 24 for number of calories per day
   burned at rest: 1,272
4. Multiply by .30 and add the result: 1,654

This is your average calorie recommendation per day.

Do not attempt to boost your BMR with chemicals or hormones. It doesn't work, and these substances can be dangerous to your health. The sensible method is through physical exercise. As the chart below demonstrates, it is difficult to expend energy without engaging in relatively vigorous activity.

ACTIVITY LEVEL	ACTIVITY	CALORIES PER MINUTE (MALE)	CALORIES PER MINUTE (FEMALE)
Sedentary	Resting in bed	1.2	1.1
	Watching TV	1.5	1.4
	Sitting	1.4	1.25

ACTIVITY LEVEL	ACTIVITY	CALORIES PER MINUTE (MALE)	CALORIES PER MINUTE (FEMALE)
	Eating	1.6	1.45
	Standing	1.6	1.45
Light activity	Sweeping floor	1.8	1.65
	Desk work	2.5	2.2
	Cooking	3.0	2.8
	Taking shower	3.8	3.4
	Walking in house	3.5	3.8
Moderate activity	Dancing	4.0	3.6
	Chopping wood	5.0	4.8
	Housekeeping	5.2	4.8
	Playing golf	5.5	5.0
Vigorous activity	Scrubbing floors	6.0	5.5
	Fast walking (4 miles/hour)	6.5	6.0
	Snow shoveling	7.0	6.8
	Tennis	7.0	6.8

ACTIVITY LEVEL	ACTIVITY	CALORIES PER MINUTE (MALE)	CALORIES PER MINUTE (FEMALE)
	Bike riding	8.0	7.8
	Heavy manual labor	7.5	7.3
Strenuous activity	Swimming	11.0	10.8
	Jogging (5 to 6 miles/hour)	18.0 to 20.0	18.0 to 20.0
	Climbing stairs	20.0	20.0

You can engage in sedentary activities indefinitely, but as the level of activity increases, you will become tired if you are not already in shape. Proper training helps establish a tolerance for higher levels of activity.

Body Fat Is Not the Enemy

As uncomfortable as most people are with the word *fat,* it is important to understand the function of adipose (fat) tissue. Fat acts as a storehouse of energy, and insures the smooth, uninterrupted delivery of valuable calories to the vital organs of our bodies. Without a fat storage system, we would be vulnerable to even a momentary lack of nutrition. Nature's genius is present in this marvelous backup.

Adipose tissue also serves other functions. As warm-blooded creatures, humans need to maintain a set temperature, and fat tissue acts as an efficient insulation system. It conserves calories in periods of energy drain.

Obese individuals, who have a thick layer of adipose tissue, lose less heat and conserve more calories than lean people. The result is that they have a harder time losing weight. Also, women have more total body fat than men, allowing them to retain heat more efficiently but have more difficulty losing weight.

BLOOD SUGAR FACT AND FICTION

Jennifer, a twenty-nine-year-old computer software program-mer, came to seek my help to lose weight. A pretty mother of two, Jennifer was at a loss in handling her intense sugar cravings. She felt the cravings were undermining her efforts.

As we talked, I learned that Jennifer had always been a hearty eater, and she came from a family of hearty eaters. Her parents and siblings all tended to be on the plump side, but this had never bothered them. "My mother believed in eating plenty of food to keep the body strong," she told me. "In fact, our family's motto was, 'A little fat on the body is good for the soul.' My mother always warned me that if I tried to diet to look skinny, I could harm myself. I bought into it, and, frankly, I've never thought much about my weight until now."

"That's interesting," I observed. "You grew up in a house-hold with a very strong and positive message about food and nourishment. It seemed to work for you. What happened to make you suddenly so desperate to lose weight?"

Jennifer flushed with embarrassment. "Last week, my hus-band, Ed, took me shopping. The sales tax on clothing was waived for a few days, and we decided to take advantage of the discount to buy clothes for the family."

Jennifer picked a few items for her children and Ed. Then she selected several items for herself and asked Ed to hold them while she quickly tried on one outfit to see if it fit. She was shocked to hear Ed say, "Honey, you picked up the wrong size on these clothes. They're size 16, not 12, like you usually wear." Jennifer realized that Ed had no clue that in the past three years she had moved up to a size 16. Not knowing what to say to him, she just returned the outfits and said, "You're right. I don't see anything I like in a size 12. Let's go."

That incident was a rude awakening for Jennifer, and at that moment she vowed to get back to a size 12. To lose weight she decided to eat cereal and orange juice for breakfast in place of pancakes, boiled eggs, and bagels with cream cheese, a light lunch in the office, and a small dinner in the evening, with no snacks before bedtime. For two days she felt wonderful, but by the third day she began to feel light-headed and weak.

Being a woman of action, Jennifer sought professional advice. She consulted a nutritionist who told her that cutting down on food had radically depleted her blood sugar, and that was why she felt so weak. He advised her to eat more food to keep the blood sugar within normal range. To Jennifer's horror, the nutritionist also warned her that she should not let her blood sugar drop drastically, as it may cause brain damage. She was scared by his comments and went back to her normal eating routine. She sought my help not knowing how to handle her body's sugar cravings.

After listening to Jennifer's story, I considered what I could do for her. Her assertion that she had low blood sugar, which could potentially become dangerous, seemed suspect to me. I doubted that she fully understood the glucose regulatory system of her body.

It is a common misconception that if you skip a meal or cut down on calories, your blood sugar will plummet. Jennifer's nutritionist was correct in saying that low blood sugar is harmful to the body, but it would never happen in a normal healthy individual, especially a person who wears a size 16.

Blood glucose is the designated fuel that supplies the body's energy needs, and its regulation is one of the most efficient systems in our body. There is a long list of supportive elements like glycogen and lipids that would never allow the blood sugar levels to be depleted, unless an individual suffers from an endocrine or metabolic disorder.

Blood tests proved that Jennifer's blood sugar was normal. Were her dizzy spells and sluggishness all in her mind? It seemed to me that there was a fairly simple explanation. For most of her life, Jennifer had eaten three good meals and snacked several times during the day. All of a sudden she threw her body into a frenzy by eating less over longer intervals. The stomach, digestive juices, and the autonomic nervous system, which controls the propulsion operation of the stomach and colon, were prepared to receive food at frequent intervals. When this did not happen, the rapidly contracting empty stomach and a slight drop in the heart rate during the time when Jennifer normally ate made her uncomfortable. If she had continued to eat less for a few more days, her body would have acclimated to the new eating routine and she would not have felt any discomfort.

DON'T BLAME YOUR GENES

Bad genes are among the reasons people use as an excuse to justify lack of control over their eating habits. For instance, Sandra, a thirty-two-year-old obese female, sought my help in losing weight. I could see that she didn't have much confidence in herself, and she confirmed my observation by saying that the genes she inherited from her parents condemned her to remain obese for the rest of her life. She was chubby as a child and obese as an adult. Her parents and older sister were all heavy. Both parents suffered from type 2 diabetes, and her father had suffered a stroke a couple of years ago. Sandra's doctor told her she had to lose at least ninety pounds to avoid the same fate as her parents.

"I don't know how to do it," she told me. "The very air I breathe seems to put on weight. Dieting has the opposite effect with me. The more I diet, the more I gain."

At one point, Sandra had given up altogether, believing that her past attempts to lose weight resulted in her gaining more weight, so she was better off not thinking of dieting at all. However, she could not stay on the sidelines any longer. The impending health crisis was too real.

I concurred with Sandra that she was probably right about her gene pool. Unfortunately, a small percentage of people are born with low BMRs. In addition, there is a great deal of individual variation when it comes to the actual physical structure of the body and its energy needs. For reasons unbeknownst to us, some people need less energy to keep their bodies healthy. Because there are no set rules as to how many calories each individual burns on a daily basis under similar physical and mental conditions, one has to figure out the calories they burn by trial and error. Besides the variation in caloric needs, there is a great deal of diversity when it comes to the total number of fat cells and their distribution throughout the body. If an individual inherits a low BMR and a higher percentage of fat cells, he or she will never be pencil thin but can work to maintain health and fitness.

The third factor that can change the energy dynamics is the

starvation syndrome. This syndrome usually remains dormant and is triggered when an individual embarks upon a highly restrictive diet to lose weight. The body does not know the individual is intentionally withholding food; it responds as if it is starving and begins to conserve energy to secure its survival. I determined that Sandra was triggering the starvation syndrome every time she dieted. Her only safe, sane, and effective course of action would be to gradually cut down on calories while slowly increasing her physical exercise.

When I explained this to Sandra, she frowned. "At that rate, it will take me two or three years to lose this weight."

"Possibly," I agreed. "But let's take a reality check. When you go on restrictive low-calorie diets to lose weight more quickly, what happens?"

"I end up gaining weight," she replied.

"And when you do nothing at all, what happens?"

"I stay the same," she said.

"Right," I said. "I am offering you a third option—to summon the patience to eat right for life, with the understanding that you will gradually lose weight and get healthier. There is no fourth option."

UNDERSTAND THE CONCEPT OF HEALTHY WEIGHT

Our society's extreme weight consciousness has created a warped sense of what it means to be overweight, underweight, or normal weight. Most people think they're overweight—that is, they could stand to lose a few pounds. However, a distorted view of what your body should look like, based on false standards of fashion models or movie stars, will only lead to frustration. You must seek a lifetime healthy weight, not a momentary fashion statement.

It was once relatively simple to find your right weight, using the old standard height/weight charts. But these charts had some major flaws. First, they did not adjust for the natural body changes that come with age. More significantly, they did not focus on healthy weight. An athlete or a bodybuilder may weigh more than the standard, but he or she may have healthier weights by virtue of muscle mass.

Many experts suggest eliminating altogether weight standards that rely on pounds. The National Institutes of Health (NIH) recommends two measurements that don't require a scale, yet they will tell you more than your scale about the shape you're in.

The first is body mass index (BMI). This is a number calculated from your weight and height that roughly correlates to the percentage of your total weight that comes from fat, as opposed to muscle, bone, or organ. The higher your BMI, the higher the percentage of fat in your body. If your BMI is under 20, you might be underweight. Between 20 and 25, you are probably at a good healthy weight for your height. A BMI over 25 is considered overweight, and over 35, obese.

The chart below will give you an estimate of your BMI. Find the intersection of your height and weight, then check the number running along the top of the chart.

The second measurement recommended by the NIH is Waist Circumference. This measurement reflects abdominal obesity, believed to be a significant factor in weight-related heart disease and diabetes.

The easiest way to measure yourself at home is by measuring your waistline at the level of the navel or at the narrowest waist midpoint using a tape measure. A woman with a waist circumference over 35 inches, or a man with a waist circumference

Body Mass Index Chart																
	19	20	21	22	23	24	25	26	27	28	29	30	31	32	33	34	35
Height (inches)	Body Weight (pounds)																
58	91	96	100	105	110	115	119	124	129	134	138	143	148	153	158	162	167
59	94	99	104	109	114	119	124	128	133	138	143	148	153	158	163	168	173
60	97	102	107	112	118	123	128	133	138	143	148	153	158	163	168	174	179
61	100	106	111	116	122	127	132	137	143	148	153	158	164	169	174	180	185
62	104	109	115	120	126	131	136	142	147	153	158	164	169	175	180	186	191
63	107	113	118	124	130	135	141	146	152	158	163	169	175	180	186	191	197
64	110	116	122	128	134	140	145	151	157	163	169	174	180	186	192	197	204
65	114	120	126	132	138	144	150	156	162	168	174	180	186	192	198	204	210
66	118	124	130	136	142	148	155	161	167	173	179	186	192	198	204	210	216
67	121	127	134	140	146	153	159	166	172	178	185	191	198	204	211	217	223
68	125	131	138	144	151	158	164	171	177	184	190	197	203	210	216	223	230
69	128	135	142	149	155	162	169	176	182	189	196	203	209	216	223	230	236
70	132	139	146	153	160	167	174	181	188	195	202	209	216	222	229	236	243
71	136	143	150	157	165	172	179	186	193	200	208	215	222	229	236	243	250
72	140	147	154	162	169	177	184	191	199	206	213	221	228	235	242	250	258
73	144	151	159	166	174	182	189	197	204	212	219	227	235	242	250	257	265
74	148	155	163	171	179	186	194	202	210	218	225	233	241	249	256	264	272
75	152	160	168	176	184	192	200	208	216	224	232	240	248	256	264	272	279
76	156	164	172	180	189	197	205	213	221	230	238	246	254	263	271	279	287

over 40 inches, is carrying too much fat around the abdominal organs.

DON'T PLAY THE DIETING GAME

If you are reading this book, I'd be willing to bet that you've been on many diets in the past. If you think of my approach as a diet, you will fail.

The typical diet plan is a two-step process. The first step is a restricted eating plan of some kind. It almost doesn't matter what kind of plan it is. Most weight-loss diets are restrictive enough in the early stages so that people lose weight. The second step of the typical diet is the maintenance plan—that is, the method of keeping the weight off. It sounds so simple, but it is so deceptive.

Most dieters are eager to embrace the first step of the diet plan, as long as they can quickly lose their excess weight. This is not hard to do. Dieters marvel at being able to lose ten or even twenty pounds in the first couple of weeks of a diet. They enthusiastically recommend the diet to their friends, and everyone signs on. But if you were to talk to these same people two or three months down the road, you would see disappointment and resentment. That's because the initial weight loss is mostly attributed to water loss, which occurs at a rapid rate. Eventually, the body reaches a critical point where it can no longer afford to lose any more water, and it begins to conserve water. Suddenly, the scale is tilting upward. Furthermore, actual fat loss occurs at a glacial pace. It is impossible to quickly lose pounds of fat.

The failure to lose weight is certainly one problem of fad diets. However, the health consequences are worse. A crash diet is like bungee jumping with a defective cord. The sudden drastic drop in calorie intake creates metabolic chaos, nutritional imbalance, and lifestyle disruption. The body literally goes into shock as the nutritional equilibrium is upset. Because the body's hormonal system (insulin, glycogen, and various enzymes that control the metabolism of carbohydrates, fats, and proteins) needs time to adjust to an alteration of nutritional status, twenty to thirty hours into a crash diet, glucose and liver glycogen reserves are completely depleted. The body needs time to generate adequate quantities of fat-dissolving enzymes to produce energy from its fat reserves. Until such time, the body attacks protein reserves and muscle glycogen to obtain energy for survival. In the interest of protecting the body from starvation, many nonvital functions are shut off.

Within a few weeks, the crash dieter is faced with the following inevitabilities:

1. The disgruntled emotional drive, deprived of pleasure, starts pressing to have its cravings met. It is often strong enough to convince the dieter to stray—or, in the lingo of dieters, to "cheat" on the diet.
2. Most of the time, crash diets suffer from nutritional myopia. As key nutrients become depleted, the dieter becomes weak and literally drained of energy.
3. As the body's metabolism slows down to conserve energy, weight loss slows to a trickle, and there may even be weight *gain,* caused by bloating. Actual fat loss becomes nearly impossible.

The sad part is that once a person stops dieting, he or she will gain back the weight that was lost, and sometimes even more. Even with a moderate calorie intake, the sluggish metabolic state will guarantee a remarkably quick return to square one.

If you have a history of dieting, you know that everything I'm saying is true. Make a choice to get off the futile dieting roller coaster and address your eating habit once and for all.

STEP 4

Make the Change

A SERIOUS EFFORT to stop overeating for good will not happen overnight. Think of it as a process that will become easier with time. In effect, you will be deprogramming your old eating habits and reprogramming your new eating habits. Your Overeating Profile will play a role in this process. I have found that different drives tend to assert themselves more vigorously at various stages and in different ways.

The following is a general idea of what you will encounter during the first few months of making this dramatic change, along with some advice for combating the emotional drives that trigger your overeating behavior.

STAGE 1: THE FIRST WEEK

Don't be surprised or dismayed if you can't get food off your mind in the first week. Eating has been the emotional core of your being for so long, that it's habitual to reach for food if you're bored, stressed, angry, happy—whenever. You may also feel real hunger as your body adapts to eating less than it is used to.

Factor in Your Overeating Profile

During the first week, the Deprivation Drive and the Insecurity Drive are the most prominent, so you need to be vigilant if your scores for these drives showed an imbalance.

The Deprivation Drive will provoke an insatiable desire to fill the void you once filled with constant overeating. Anticipate feelings of deprivation, and prepare to address them. Think about the times of day that are most difficult for you, and schedule a change in your routine. For example, if your regular routine is to sit in front of the TV and snack, make the TV off-limits for a week, or incorporate an activity, like folding laundry or paying bills while you watch your favorite program. You can also work out or walk on a treadmill while you watch TV.

You can minimize the effects of the Deprivation Drive by making sure you are not physically depriving your body of needed calories. I recommend keeping track of calories in your journal. This helps establish a discipline; it also reminds you that you are getting sufficient calories and that your appetite pangs are emotional, not physical, signals.

It will also help to be more intentional about the way you eat. I have noticed that many obese people do not chew their food properly, and they eat very fast, as if it were their last meal. Without paying attention to what we eat and taking the time to enjoy it, we may never derive full pleasure and satisfaction from food and, therefore, feel deprived. It is a vicious circle. The additional advantage of eating slowly is that there is enough time for your stomach to alert you to the right moment to stop eating.

If you have dieted many times in the past and always failed, your Insecurity Drive will be in high gear, planting seeds of doubt that you can succeed this time. Your journal will help here, too. Write down what you are feeling. Articulate your fears, and then articulate your resolve. It will help. You may also benefit by joining a group. I often find that people with a strong Insecurity Drive benefit from Weight Watchers or similar programs. It boosts their courage to see that others are in the same boat and are determined to succeed.

STAGE 2: FROM TWO TO SIX WEEKS

After you've made it through the first week, your level of confidence will be higher as you see that you're capable of controlling your cravings. You will also begin to experience some positive physical rewards. Your body will have adjusted to the new eating pattern, and you'll probably be feeling more energy. Regular physical exercise will also increase your energy and make you feel stronger. You may be amazed the first time you realize that you aren't experiencing your usual midday sluggishness.

You will also experience a small but steady weight loss. This will be pleasing, but you may also be frustrated that you are not losing more weight faster. Let me strongly emphasize this point: you may lose several pounds in the first week or two, but this will primarily be water weight. Healthy, long-term weight loss should stay in the range of half a pound to one pound a week. If you are losing more, you are not eating sufficient calories, or you are exercising too strenuously. This sets you up for the starvation syndrome, which will reverse your hard work. Have patience and stay on course.

Factor in Your Overeating Profile

During this period, the Entitlement Drive and the Defiant Drive are the most prominent, so you need to be vigilant if your scores for these drives showed an imbalance.

As the weeks progress, you may find yourself living with a tempting and taunting idea that you should reward yourself for all of your hard work by splurging on your favorite foods. The Entitlement Drive can poke at your resolve like a spoiled child crying for a lollipop after a doctor's visit. Be ready with small rewards that don't involve food. For example, after a stressful day at work, treat yourself to a massage or a swim at the pool. Make a date to see a movie. Call a friend.

You can also short-circuit the Entitlement Drive by scheduling a treat every week—such as a Sunday dessert or a slice of pizza with friends. If your emotional drives are in check, you need not worry that one treat will set you off on a bingeing escapade. Remember, appetite is emotional, not physical. You can control it.

If the Defiant Drive has been a factor in your eating behavior, you may find it making a return visit as the weeks go by. In response to your discomfort, you may be tempted to say, "I don't have to put up with this misery. I'll do what I want." Instead, turn your defiance on your habit, making it work for you, not against you. Say, "I refuse to let a hamburger run my life." You may be helped by joining a group where you can articulate your strong feelings in a supportive environment.

STAGE 3: FROM SIX WEEKS TO THREE MONTHS

Although your body's metabolism has adjusted to your new routine, and you are enjoying many physical and emotional benefits, you need to be on the alert for a false sense of confidence. The holidays or a vacation can thwart your progress. Such occasions trigger an automatic craving for certain foods and eating patterns. For example, many of my patients live in dread of Thanksgiving. They can practically taste the rich gravy, the chestnut stuffing, and mom's pumpkin pie in their minds. Not only do they long for these foods, which are associated with positive family memories, but they know they will constantly be pressured to indulge. I tell them that the best defense is a good offense. Neutralize the craving by eating a small snack before the big meal. Spare Mom's feelings by having a tiny slice of pie. It's in your control.

During this period, you will not constantly feel the temptation to overeat, but you must have vigilance. A trivial, disappointing incident immediately triggers a need to be comforted. That's fine. Look for comfort, but vow that food no longer represents comfort to you.

Factor in Your Overeating Profile

During this period, the Disenchantment Drive and the Invincibility Drive are the most prominent, so you need to be vigilant if your scores for these drives showed an imbalance.

The Disenchantment Drive provokes memories of your former pleasures, which may be strong at times, accompanied by a sense of loss of a good friend, followed by sadness. You may be touchy and sensitive. Rather than basking in your sadness, work to create a more pleasing environment. Physical exercise can help here. Exercise is a natural mood lifter.

The Invincibility Drive can be the hardest to conquer. The very fact that you have exerted the patience and discipline to pursue your goals can trigger a renewed sense of invincibility.

You may feel that because you have succeeded, it's not so hard to change whenever you want to. You're in control. You can gain a pound or two without worry. Don't allow these self-deceptive notions to creep in on you. Remember, your aim is not just to lose weight or temporarily curb your diet. You are embarking on a journey to maintain a healthy weight for the remainder of your life.

STAGE 4: FROM THREE MONTHS TO SIX MONTHS

If you have a history of yo-yo dieting, this period is probably foreign terrain for you. Few fad diets last more than a few weeks before the poor misled dieter cries uncle. After the third month, your routine should be starting to feel less like a program and more like a lifestyle.

LEARN THE ART OF EATING RIGHT

There are no simple or easy ways to satisfy the needs of both the mind and body without compromising the laws of nature. Either the mind or body, or at times both, will have to compromise for the greater good. Therefore, it is an art to balance the needs of both to maintain everlasting peace of mind, good health, and security.

Eating right is an art, not a science. For example, knowing the nutritional value of food will certainly help you know how to eat right. But the knowledge must be combined with the inborn instincts and creativity that are the human birthright. A world-class musician has to be born with a musical talent. Without that strong foundation the learned musical knowledge alone will not create a musical genius. Therefore an individual has to practice eating right and managing weight properly like an art, not a science.

The laws of nature expect our minds to put the nutritional needs of our bodies before our likes and dislikes. If we follow nature's cues in deciding what to eat, when to eat, where to eat, and how much to eat, eating right will become an art, not a science. I assure you that if you have the right attitude about your diet, you will make good choices even if you know very little about nutrition.

For me, eating right, keeping my weight stable, and staying healthy is an art, not a science, because I have assured my body that I will never put my wants before its needs. I have always taken good care of my body and I consider it my top duty. My body is my best friend, not my worst enemy. If I viewed my body as my enemy, I could have eaten gallons of chocolate ice cream and banana cream pies every day. Why not? It is a mandate to defeat one's enemies.

Instead, I have embraced my body as a friend. I take care of its nutritional needs first, and then turn to my emotional needs and satisfy them only when it will do no harm. It is definitely an art to achieve a balance between the mind's want and the body's needs. When I choose not to eat certain food at certain times, I do not feel deprived and therefore it becomes an effortless task. I certainly select foods that I enjoy the most, but I make sure that they are not harmful to my body.

Finally, I have made a vow to never eat when I am stressed, bored, happy, or sad. I take my daily tasks as challenges not as chores, and therefore I have practically eliminated the stress in my life. Even when I experience tough times, I know that eating more food will compound my problems, not resolve them. Therefore, when my patients tell me they overeat because they are sad or disenchanted, I always ask them if food solved their problems. They look at me sheepishly and concede that it did not. They overeat as a consolation, not as a solution to their problem, but they are not consoled. It's quite an eye-opener when they recognize this.

How to Eat

You are an individual, and what works best for one person will not necessarily work for you. I am not a dietician, and you will find no lists of foods or dieting rules in this book. For that, you have hundreds of books and Web sites at your disposal. The following suggestions are very broad guidelines. I encourage you to make regular use of the journal sheets in the appendix to chart your progress, plan your meals, and reflect on your life's journey.

How Many Calories?

Begin by calculating the total number of calories your body needs each day. Use the BMR calculation on pages 83 and 84 as a guide, adding or subtracting according to your physical activity and desired weight loss.

When and How Often?

Next, determine the number of times you wish to eat in a day, and how you are going to use your calories. Be realistic. Consider your schedule, obligations, time for food preparation, etc. For example, one of my patients was a salesman who was on airplanes three or four days a week. He correctly determined that a diet of airplane food would eventually be his downfall, so he trained himself to eat a small meal when he got up in the morning, and then eat nothing but fruit until late in the afternoon. His eating schedule looked like this:

Early morning: 25 percent of total
Fruit/nuts during the day: 15 percent of total
Late afternoon soup or salad: 25 percent of total
Evening meal: 35 percent of total

Decide how you will allot your calories. Contrary to popular belief, there is no measurable difference in weight loss if you avoid calories in the evening and eat more calories in the morning. If you are eating approximately the same amount every day, your body will adjust. It's more important for you to devise a schedule that is comfortable for you, and that determination is more complicated than biological considerations. The key is balance. Your goal is to avoid situations when extreme hunger might tempt you to grab a fast-food meal or snack.

With time, you will develop an instinct for the right mix. For example, I eat fewer calories than my body needs for five days a week. I eat a little more on the weekends. In a sense, I lose a little bit of weight from Monday through Friday and gain a little bit of weight on the weekend. I am very much used to my regular weight. Even if I gain one pound I feel sluggish. However, you must treat any weight gain, even one pound, as if it were twenty pounds. If you do not take the first pound of weight gain seriously, then you will lose the battle of the bulge. If you are not careful, the pounds will sneak up on you and before you notice, you will have accumulated ten to fifteen pounds.

This advice is for healthy individuals. If you have health conditions that require you to eat more frequently, consult your physician for guidance.

What Foods?

What should you eat? As I have pointed out, I am not a dietician. There are many references that can educate you in proper nutritional balance—including the Food Pyramid. On a very basic level, make sure your diet includes a healthy balance of carbohydrates (especially complex carbohydrates found in fruits, vegetables, and whole grains), protein, and fat (especially unsaturated fat).

Here is a technique I've found to be effective: List all the food items that you like to eat, and divide the list into two categories. The first category should contain more volume, fewer calories, but adequate amounts of vegetables, whole grains and rice, beans and legumes, nuts and oil, fruit, low-fat/nonfat dairy, seafood (except for crustaceans), white meat and lean red meats. Choose solely from this group on a daily basis.

The second list should contain foods that you enjoy, but are not necessary for your health. These foods appeal to your psyche more than your body. Put anything you like on the list, and choose one item every week or two for a special occasion.

I'm sure many nutritional purists would scoff at this recommendation. They would suggest banning milk shakes and sausage patties altogether. The reason I am not troubled by an occasional treat is because I realize that, in control, the pleasure derived from food can be positive. Furthermore, once you are on a healthy eating plan, your tastes and cravings may change completely. Having addressed your emotional cravings, you are not in danger of falling off the wagon with a bite of cream puff. Indeed, there is no longer any wagon to fall off!

Exercise, Exercise, Exercise

There are no two ways about it. You must exercise in order to be fit, and it is virtually impossible to lose weight if your plan does not have an exercise component. This should be your mantra to be slim, trim, healthy, and energetic for the rest of your life.

Unless you diligently follow the workout plan you laid out for yourself, you will never be able to correct your overeating habit. Any gap in your exercise plan will be the first sign of a weakened resolve, and eventually your overeating habits will return. If anyone believes that they can maintain proper weight forever without physically working out, they are fooling themselves. You cannot be physically lazy and remain slim, trim, and healthy. Thanks (or no thanks!) to the marvels of modern technology, it is impossible to get enough physical exercise by doing your job (unless you're a manual laborer or an athlete) or by housekeeping. You have to make an effort. Here's a case in point. One of my patients, an executive in New York City, wanted to lose weight and he complained that he didn't have time to go to a gym. He took the train to the city every day from his home in the suburbs, so I asked him how far it was from his house to the train station. He measured the distance; it was one and one quarter miles. "How long is the drive?" I asked. He said it took between seven and eight minutes. I suggested that he start walking back and forth to the station instead of driving, and see what happened.

He was enthusiastic about my suggestion, and within two months he was able to walk the distance in eighteen minutes. The addition of a two-and-a-half-mile walk each workday allowed him to quickly lose a few pounds. And he reported feeling better than ever.

I often suggest to patients who work in office buildings that they take the stairs instead of the elevator. At a calorie expenditure rate of 20 calories per minute, stair-climbing is one of the most effective exercises there is. It can also be faster than the elevator. I work in a hospital that has six floors, and I rarely use the elevators. In the course of nineteen years, the stairs and I have become very good friends. I am faster than any elevator service. It amuses me that some people will wait five minutes or more for an elevator that is only taking them to the next floor.

Use the journal pages in the Appendix to plan your exercise regimen and record your progress. If you're not used to exercising, start slow, with a goal of working up to thirty minutes a day, six days a week, or forty-five minutes a day, five days a week.

Walking is the cheapest, easiest, and most effective exercise plan. It's also something almost everyone can do. You don't need a gym membership, fancy equipment, or exercise videos—just a pair of good walking shoes.

The best time to exercise is first thing in the morning. If that is not possible, lunchtime at work is acceptable. But you should try to avoid an exercise program that involves working out in the evenings. In my experience, there are too many loopholes after a long day of work. These include: simple exhaustion, stress, hunger, family obligations, phone calls, and social engagements. Any of these can sidetrack you from your routine.

Minutes Needed for the Body to Burn Calories					
FOOD	CALORIES	SITTING	GOLFING	WALKING (4 MILES/ HOUR)	STAIR CLIMBING
med. orange	65	46	12	10	3
med. banana	90	64	16	14	4
large apple	100	71	18	15	5
med. potato	100	71	18	15	5
½ cup spinach	20	14	4	3	1
med. boiled egg	80	57	15	12	4
1 pork chop	310	220	56	48	15
8 oz. whole milk	165	119	30	25	8
doughnut	150	107	27	23	7.5
8 oz. beer	115	82	21	18	5
chocolate milk shake (8 oz.)	530	379	96	82	26.5

THE JOY OF EATING

I clearly remember my childhood days in India. We ate our dinner as a family at 8:00 P.M. My father sat at the head of the table with his four children on either side, all of us eagerly looking forward to being served delicious food by our loving and caring mother. I have to admit that my mother was a darn good cook. But more than remembering the food itself, my memories of our family meals are filled with the ambience of warmth and pleasure that nourished our hearts as well as our bodies.

After the main meal, my mother brought a generous platter of fruit, which we nibbled while we talked. This was the time our father asked about our days, and invited us to share our problems with him.

Because of my experience, I think I realized from a relatively early age that food alone has little to offer the psyche. If you gulp down a slice of pizza while you're busy working at your computer, you may get a brief rush of pleasure, but you will never experience the enveloping sense of contentment I recall from my family dinners.

Food should be served in a lovely and friendly environment to have a positive, permanent impact on our emotions. This type of relationship with food is necessary to develop healthy eating habits. In the absence of an inspired environment, food becomes an empty way to pacify the raw emotions without providing lasting satisfaction.

I believe our forefathers knew how to eat right. Besides the seductive environment in which they ate, they also enjoyed another distinct advantage over us. They engaged both their minds and their bodies in their work. The lack of heavy machinery, automobiles, and telephones now appears to have been a blessing in disguise. Between healthy eating habits and regular manual labor, I believe our forefathers remained healthy, trim, and fit.

The lesson I learned by observing my parents and grandparents is that I am blessed to have a job, a wonderful family, delicious home-cooked meals, and a good night's sleep. Because I am content in life, it is not so difficult to say no to my favorite foods, which include vanilla ice cream, lightly salted potato chips, lightly salted peanuts, and banana cake. I don't feel sad or deprived whenever I say no to these delicacies to protect my health, because I cherish my health more than food.

I encourage you to cherish your health. For instance, use the stairs instead of the elevators whenever possible. Walk to the local stores or train stations instead of driving. Get out of the office at lunch and take a half-hour walk with an apple in one hand and a bottle of water in the other. You will immensely benefit from this routine in more ways than one. You will be in a great mood after lunch and you will burn some calories.

STEP 5

Conquer the Dieting Mentality

MAKE NO MISTAKE about it. Being obsessed with food is a form of slavery, and your goal should be freedom. Unfortunately, the current culture of "recovery," which has extended to overeaters, promotes the idea of "once a food addict, always a food addict."

This is where I part ways with the 12-step ideology, especially as it applies to overeating. The 12-step method encourages people to think of their cravings as permanent—like dormant bombs set to explode without warning. Constant vigilance is required. In my experience, what every overeater really longs for is normalcy—a state of comfort with food, rather than fearful obsession, and the state of comfortable nonaddiction, not continued obsession. They are unwilling to spend another minute of their lives in this trap. I say they don't have to.

Through the emotional adjustment I outline in this book, most people are able to control the desire to seek comfort from food on a day-to-day basis. However, they almost always say they carry a deep dread of what will occur the first time they experience a highly stressful situation. They don't trust their instincts to choose a different, more productive method of relief— probably because they've "fallen off the wagon" so many times in the past.

If you are to be successful in conquering your enemy, you must face your past eating compulsion without fear, and know that it hasn't left a permanent tattoo on your mind.

Start today to eliminate the dieter's mentality, which saps your self-esteem and weakens your resolve. How is it accomplished? Remember, the Instinctual Division of the mind is not independent of the Intellectual and Emotional division. The instinct to reach for your favorite comfort food in times of stress is a learned behavior. Even when the Emotional Division is no longer demanding the relief, the Instinctual Division must be reconfigured to respond differently. In essence, it must be trained to have an alternative automatic response to stress.

We all face obstacles in life regularly. Sometimes we are distressed, upset, disappointed, or hurt. Being treated unfairly by others hurts us the most. Believe it or not, it happens to us all the time. Pain and anguish demand immediate compensation. We need to do something to soothe the pain at that moment of distress. We take an inventory of what activities have given or could give us relief and comfort on such occasions. Usually, addictive habits are at the top of that list, and we go for them, even if we had once parted with them. Your task will be to evaluate the other items on that list that you can use instead.

I ask my patients to perform visualization exercises—to picture themselves at the final moment when they close the door on their obsessive eating and lock it behind them. Some have difficulty looking ahead; some balk at locking the door. Some experience a sudden urge to take one last look. This exercise is immensely powerful. It completes the emotional adjustment. Closing the door, placing a sturdy lock on it, and throwing away the key, you bid farewell to your desperation and deprivation, your bitterness and fear, your insecurity and disappointment. These destructive emotional drives no longer exist for you in the realm of nourishment.

As you begin to see yourself and your place in the world in a more realistic light, these priorities will emerge naturally: peace of mind, unadulterated good health, freedom, and the natural high that comes from being at one with nature. When your priorities are straight, everything else falls into place. You may still strive to make good money, but the desire for money won't run you. You may seek material comforts, but not need them for your well-being. Your relationships will occur naturally on your own terms; you will no longer feel the need to create facades to make yourself more popular, or hide from others out of fear of rejection. You can delight in nourishing your body, along with your soul.

APPENDIX

Your Personal
Stop Overeating for Good Journal

I have provided three charts below to help you keep track of your goals and progress. Before starting, write your goals in your journal, calculating your average range of calories per day and your method and amount of exercise. Here is a brief explanation of the charts:

Daily Food Journal

Studies show that people who keep a journal of their eating behaviors are more successful achieving and maintaining a healthy weight. The reason for this is clear. Keeping a journal is an exercise in consciousness. It is a way to exert your mind over your habit.

The following journal is designed to help you maintain that control. There are six elements.

1. TIME: Strive to eat at the same times every day. I recommend that you separate your meals by at least four hours, which will help you regulate your metabolism. Your time record will show you at a glance

whether you are susceptible to spontaneous or emotional eating when you are not hungry.

2. FOOD: Your diet should include an abundance of whole grains, fruits and vegetables, and a minimum of healthy fats and animal proteins. The USDA Food Pyramid is actually a fairly good guideline for a healthy diet. If you have the right mind-set, the Food Pyramid can work for you. There are also many helpful resources through the American Heart Association and the American Diabetic Association. If you have access to the Web, you can find an abundance of menus and eating tips through these resources.

3. PORTION SIZE: I have found that most people have little idea of what a normal portion size is. Americans are used to eating in restaurants and fast-food joints, where supersizing is practiced. Get in the habit of reading the labels on packaged foods and weighing your portions on a small kitchen scale.

4. CALORIES: I recommend that you purchase an inexpensive calorie guide. If you rigorously keep track of your daily calories, you will find that it makes a big difference. You may think twice before you have that second helping. In time, it will become second nature to eat the right amounts.

5. OTHER: You may also find it useful to keep track of your daily fat or sugar intake. Or if you regularly drink alcohol, such as a glass of wine with dinner, I suggest that you cut down on this or eliminate it entirely in the beginning. Not only is alcohol high in sugar and calories, it can also weaken your discipline. Be aware of specific food and drink items that can sabotage your mental commitment.

6. REFLECTION: At the end of each day, take a moment to reflect on your eating habits for that day. Did you meet your calorie goal? Did you eat when you were bored, angry, or frustrated? What was your energy level throughout the day? What adjustments do you need to make? Restate your intention for the coming day.

Daily Exercise Journal

Here is an explanation of the categories in your daily exercise chart.

1. TIME: If possible, try to exercise at the same time every day. I believe the best time is first thing in the morning, when there is less chance of being distracted by other obligations, or when you are less likely to be tired after a long day at work. If you exercise during your lunch hour, be sure to take along some fruit and protein, such as yogurt, so you don't suffer from a depletion of blood sugar. Exercise should energize you, not exhaust you.

2. ACTIVITY: Write down the activity, even if it isn't regimented. For example, if you walk up four flights of stairs instead of taking the elevator, make a note of it.

3. LEVEL: Note whether your activity is low, moderate, or high. You can refer to the chart on pages 85 and 86 for guidelines.

4. DISTANCE/ENDURANCE: Depending on the exercise you choose, write down the endurance (amount of time), distance (if you are walking, jogging, biking, in-line skating, or swimming), and amount of weight (if you are doing strength training).

5. OTHER: Use this box to note other activities, such as a game of tennis, golf, or basketball.

6. REFLECTION: At the end of each day, take a moment to reflect on your exercise achievements for that day. Did you keep your exercise commitment? Exceed it? Did you go out of your way to be physically active when the opportunity presented itself—such as walking a few blocks instead of driving? Describe how you felt after exercising. If you did not exercise, write down the reason, and renew your commitment for the next day.

Weekly Reflection

At the end of each week, spend a half an hour or so reviewing the week. Begin by evaluating your eating and exercise charts, and writing down how many days you met your goal. What were your successes? What were your mental/emotional impediments to success? Consider the steps you can take to overcome them in the coming week.

Remember that this is not a diet plan; it is the beginning of a lifestyle you are creating. There may be stumbling blocks, but there is no failure.

DAILY FOOD JOURNAL

TIME	FOOD	PORTION	CALORIES	OTHER

Reflection:

DAILY EXERCISE JOURNAL				
TIME	ACTIVITY	LEVEL	DISTANCE/ ENDURANCE	OTHER

Reflection:

WEEKLY REFLECTION	
FOOD	
EXERCISE	
MIND–SET	

INDEX